Concussion Recovery is an extremely practical guide written from first hand experience. This thought provoking handbook with proven strategies will assist survivors and caregivers in rebuilding their lives after an accident.

~ Harry Zarins, M.Ed.
Executive Director
Brain Injury Association of Canada
Web: www.biac-aclc.ca
Twitter: http://twitter.com/biacaclc

Brain Injury Association of Canada
Association canadienne des lésés cérébraux

www.biac-aclc.ca

"*Experience is the best teacher*" certainly applies to Ms. Colleen Butler. Brain injury is far more common and much more insidious than has ever been suspected. Colleen writes from first-hand experience, in an effort to give hope, comfort and practical proposals for people going through brain injury, as well as their caregivers.

~ Dr. Kate Brooks, ND
Living Well Center, Atlanta, Georgia

I dedicate this to all the people who have fallen through the cracks and those who feel that the journey is impossible.

You are not alone. It is possible.

Your brain can be taken from you but it is yours to reclaim and rebuild.

Concussion Recovery

Contents

A Personal Welcome 5

Falling Between the Cracks: My Story 9

The Story of Reg 14

Glossary of Terms 16

Diagnostic Tools 17

The Stages of Recovery 19

Different Kinds of Recovery 22

Parts of the Brain 23

Body Structure 31

Nutrition 33

Nutritional Supplements 41

Sleep 51

Emotional Aspects 58

Post Traumatic Stress Disorder 71

Physical Exercise 74

Mental Exercise 87

Boundaries 93

Music 99

Spiritual Aspects 101

Sex and Intimacy 103

The Healing Team 105

In Closing 107

I am trillions of cells sharing a common mind.

Dr. Jill Bolte Taylor, Phd.

A Personal Welcome

Yes, you have a concussion. This is not the end of the world. However, the journey to recovery will take great strength and courage.

A part of the brain is damaged but what you need to know is exactly how much brain power you really have.

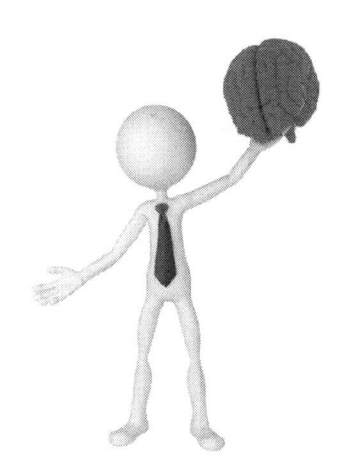

How smart are you, really?

Here is a little information to keep your injury in perspective.

- The diameter of an individual neuron is just 4 microns thick.
- 30 000 neurons can fit on the head of a pin.[i]
- Each brain cell has the equivalent capacity of a home computer.
- If you lined up all of your brain cells, they would reach from Earth to the Moon and back. That is a distance of about 700 000 kilometers![ii]

I would say you are pretty smart!

So, yes, you have an injury. But look at all of the resources you have in your brain. We just need to learn to reroute the signals so that you can regain your life. Once the correct environment has been created, the neurons can fire and start sending messages to the correct parts of your brain.

Concussion Recovery

Think of it this way... Your mind is a large city. One day, you hop in your car to go to the grocery store. Instead, you get caught in a traffic jam. You can choose to sit and wait, or you can try another route. The same choice is available when you experience a brain injury!

This book is written to show alternative routes to your destination. Together, we will get there. But we might need to make a few detours on the way!

Remember, though, that reading this is not enough to get you better. There is no magic carpet. Be an active participant and do the exercises.

Our brains are amazing. They dictate everything to us: happy or sad, hungry or satiated, tired or invigorated, hot or cold, how to move our right eyelid or wiggle our left toe.

Our brains are the motherboard in our computer. When we have a head injury, we are defragging and then rebuilding our computer. To defrag our brain, we collect all of the old ways of doing things and put them in the trash. In our recovery, we are simply uploading the newest edition of ourselves and who we want to be. We will not be exactly who we used to be. But our transformed selves will be wonderful and happy!

A head injury shakes us up enough that we become aware of different things around us and, I must admit, humbled by the elements in our world and in nature. We have the opportunity

Concussion Recovery

to learn new programs. If we fight the change, we will be stuck until we are willing to let go of old ways of thinking and doing.

Competitive people will soon learn, like I did, about patience and about honoring time to heal. Healing cannot be pushed. Each head injury or concussion is different. The area of the damage, the velocity of the hit and your health will all determine the recovery time.

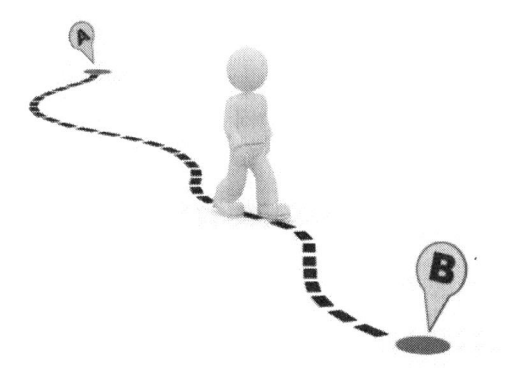

Being proactive and setting up the right environment in which to move forward is the best that can be done. If you push through 5 hours of physical or mental exercise, when 2 is what is needed, you will set yourself back. Learning to honor your body and respect its time to heal may be the most difficult thing to do.

Scientists claim that an adult needs approximately 7-10 years to completely recover from a brain injury. This estimate is pretty accurate if you are left alone to recover. But, by being proactive and progressive, recovery time can be greatly reduced.

Concussion Recovery

Of course, you will have to be a bit of your own doctor by examining your chart to know which part of the brain has been damaged, checking in with your feelings and then guiding your own recovery with good nutrition, quiet, sleep, and mental, physical and emotional exercises. Be gentle with yourself. Let this book be your toolbox.

Now let's begin.

Concussion Recovery

Falling Between the Cracks: My Story

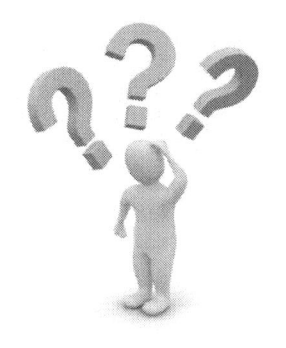

Here is a little piece of advice, which I used to offer people, especially women. I used to say, "Get smart. Get educated. That is the one thing in the world that cannot be taken from you. They can take your car and your house. You can trade in your spouse. You can lose all your money. But no one can take your brain."

Little did I know that, for the next three years, I would be eating those words.

On the day of my brain injury I was sitting on my back patio during lunch, thinking about how my life was so blessed. After all, I was fortunate enough to be able to create a vision in my head, and then make that vision into a physical reality. In a way, it was like playing dress-up. On an empty building lot, I could design and build a home, and then try out new color schemes, new kitchen and bathroom designs. Then I could sell the home and start again.

At that time, I thought life does not get much better than that!

At 1:35 pm, as I was pulling out from a side street, a fully loaded, five ton, industrial truck T-boned me and pushed my vehicle 200 feet down the road. I walked away unharmed from that accident. Or so I thought... This is where my story begins.

Concussion Recovery

(handwritten at top: "Not head injury")

Even though I had heard a snap in the right-hand side of the back of my neck, I was convinced that there was nothing wrong with me. Being self-employed, I felt that I had to get back to work.

My head was still there; there was no blood, no swelling. My vehicle was totaled. But I was fine!

Then my body and my life gradually seized up. I was present in situations but really I was nothing and did nothing. I did not understand my sudden unhappiness.

One day in particular stands out for me. I drove home for an appointment but I was not able to get out of my truck. My body refused to move. Tears ran down my face from pain and frustration. I was losing control of my life. *(handwritten: Yep)*

I remember the soreness in my back when I tried to bend over to pick up a small piece of a 2x4. Someone would say, "Hi," and I would start crying. When I was not crying, I would repeat to myself all those conversations that I was obsessed about. I could not stop. *(handwritten: Yep)*

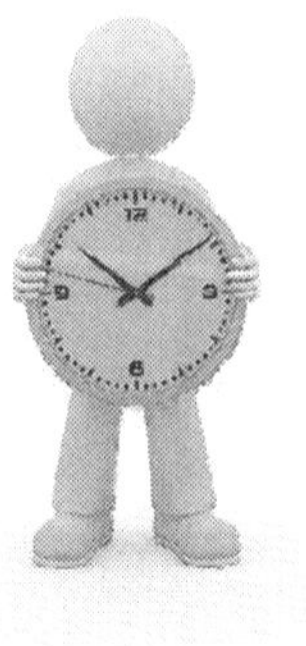

I lost all track of time. Everything in my head was mixed up. Agitated for no reason, I could not cope. My head had been shaken up so that the fluid was not circulating in my brain.

Concussion Recovery

Imagine a live electrical cord being split open and flaying around the streets in puddles of water, exploding even more. That is how my brain was misfiring. I was not connecting life with reality.

I saw a doctor. But he just touched my shoulder and told me that I might feel some soreness. That was it; no tests, no warnings. He never warned me that I might become a psycho lady!

With this loss of articulation and quick thinking, I gave my lawyer the power of attorney over me. We had simple meetings during which I would just break down and cry whenever I was asked a question. I could see mouths moving but nothing made sense. Simple business became 100 percent overwhelming.

Really, life was pretty overwhelming for those first two years. I started to doubt myself because of all of the talk that was going on in my head. A whirlwind of confusion and of lost self-confidence, I didn't know what was happening. It was scary.

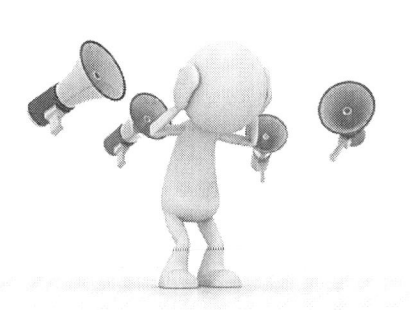

Being a relatively proud person, I kept things hidden. I stayed home and only did what was absolutely essential. No one knew my dark thoughts. It was as if I lived behind a set of sheer

Concussion Recovery

curtains. Happy or sad, my emotions became neutral. Life was passing me by.

Of course, along with this, sleep deprivation made things even worse. When I could not sleep, I would get up and watch old slow running movies. Old movies became my sedative.

My state was not conducive to my highly demanding job where, at any given time, there might be 10 people waiting for me to tell them how to keep their teams of people going. I needed to be on top of my game, quick-witted, fast thinking and articulate. But, in reality, I was a blundering babbling empty shell.

Rumors about me flew around like wild fire. I could keep things together if they were on my time, in my time. But with any pressure, I would explode in frustration and become so overwhelmed. The juices of life that fed me before the accident had become my poison! — plus meds,

In one hour, I went from walking to not being able to move my legs or arms at all. They would stay seized up for 24-30 hours. Not only would I cry on the spot, but I could not handle the slightest conflict or stress. I was often physically unable to move.

People were quick to pass judgment on me. Some of the friends I had known before the accident could no longer stand to be around me. They could not understand why I am so different

Concussion Recovery

now because there was no cast on my head to identify my damaged thinking. *Told um not different* ~~Yes~~

I was tired all the time. Yet sleep did not help my exhaustion. The doctors called it 'depression.' No kidding! I could no longer join the dots of life and I was looking for a bridge to jump off. I had gone from 120 mph to reverse in slow motion. The doctors offered no answers. I had completely fallen between the cracks. My regular doctor said, *"This just happens with accidents. It is the stress. Here, take some Prozac."* — *too many meds*

My first sign of relief came when I read the book, *My Stroke of Insight*, which emphasizes this truth: Sleep relaxes the brain when it goes into overload. You need sleep to rest the brain. Wow, that was a day of freedom! *(e.g. Sisalet)*

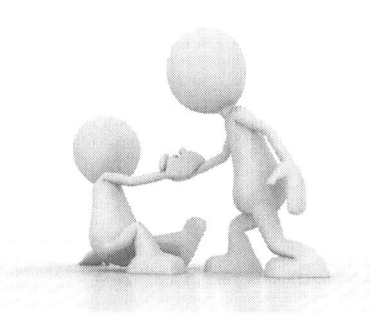

I started to seek help. A chiropractor started with the alignment of my body. There were a few people who really got me through those days, one leading to the other. I kept looking for the right person. But then I realized that I was the right person. Then the rebuilding began. Life is precious and should be treasured. We never know what is around the corner or what tomorrow will bring. All we have is the present.

My struggle does not need to be duplicated.

Concussion Recovery

I believe that to have knowledge and not share it is perhaps the largest sin. So this is my gift to you. May this book help you along your journey to recovery.

The Story of Reg

Let me tell you about a dear friend of mine, named Reg, who hit his head 35 years ago when the logging truck he was driving skidded off a dock, dropped 30 feet into the ocean, and then plummeted another 30 feet to the ocean floor. He was rescued, spent a week in the hospital and was released.

There was never a discussion of the possibility of a brain injury or concussion.

Shortly thereafter, he re-trained as a welder, made a mistake and received burns to approximately 75 percent of his body.

With the responsibility of a young family, he took up the trade of dry walling and appeared to be very successful on the surface. Reg was an exceptional worker with a great team. You would think his life was perfect.

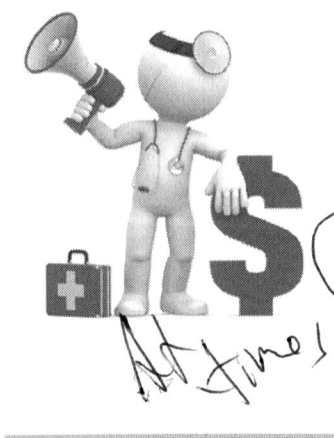

Managing money and completing tasks in a timely matter are keys to surviving in business. Reg could not manage his money or his time, and alcohol became his coping mechanism. Bankruptcy was

Concussion Recovery

inevitable.

Thirty-five struggling years have passed since the accident. Reg has lived with the constant grogginess of drugs that were prescribed by his doctor.

After three bankruptcies, help finally arrived and Reg began the process of rebuilding his brain, his life and his family. One of his most difficult tasks was getting off the drugs, which he had taken for three-quarters of his life. It has been an uphill battle.

Everything we know about the brain has been discovered within the last 10 years. This is new territory. In fact, Reg told me that his dog helped him heal more than all of his doctors and the results of the medical tests.

Please be vigilant in your recovery. Challenge the knowledge that is presented to you. With a head injury, you have to guide those who are helping you the best you can. You are your own best advocate.

Glossary of Terms

What is a head injury? A head injury is a hit, bang, jar or impact to the head, which affects the brain.

What is a brain injury? A brain injury occurs as a result of the brain hitting the inside of the skull. The brain may rip, tear, bruise or break open within the skull. Internal bleeding may or may not occur. The stationary structure of the skull does not expand. The pressure from internal bleeding may be fatal if the skull is not opened to relieve the pressure.

What is a concussion? A concussion is a brain injury. A concussion may result from one or multiple hits to the head. The effects may be experienced immediately or they may be unveiled after weeks or months. There may be exterior swelling as well. Bleeding may or may not occur.

ABI: Acquired Brain Injuries (ABI) are injuries to the brain that occur from one or more impacts. ABI`s are rated mild to severe.

TBI: Traumatic Brain Injuries (TBI) are more intense than ABI. The patient may be in a coma and may have to relearn the basic skills of walking, talking, eating etc. TBI`s are rated mild to severe.

Coup and contra coup brain contusion is an internal whiplash of the brain. It occurs when the head is jolted in one direction. The brain is pushed in the direction of the jolt, hits the inside of the skull, and then bounces back. The side of the brain opposite to the accident is damaged.

Diagnostic Tools

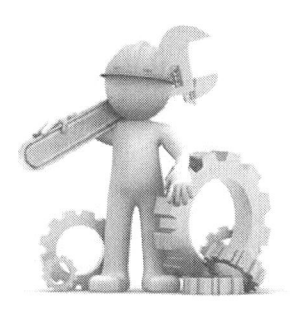

The world's leading scientists recognize that no machine can accurately detect or predict the severity of a brain injury. Andrew R. Mayer, PhD, is a research scientist at the Mind Research Network in Albuquerque, NM. He admits that, "*One of the frustrating problems in patients with mild traumatic brain injury is that conventional neuroimaging doesn't show anything.*"

In our age of technological prowess, this is almost unbelievable. Yet we still want to place our hope in medical tests and even wait for months like laboratory rats for the results.

Each head injury is unique and there is nothing outside of your own head with which to diagnose the nature and severity of it. We need to become aware of our environment and our bodies.

Yes, we need to respond to all that 'touchy feely' stuff that we have pushed to the side. If you have maintained a stiff upper lip, it may have taken a hit on the head to wake you up and open you up to the feeling side of the brain.

Brain injuries have a journey of their own, a time of their own and gifts to give. You will get in touch with yourself in a way that you have never experienced and, during the journey, you

Concussion Recovery

may consider including modern medicine as a tool in your healing tool box.

At the present time, modern medicine offers these options:

- **X-Ray** will only show bone fractures as brains are jellied mass.
- **CT Scan** is only a more sophisticated X-Ray.
- **MRI Function/ Resting state** records the structure of how the brain works.
- **EEG: electroencephalograph** measures electrical movement in the brain like seizures and sleep patterns.
- **PET Scan: Positive Emission Tomography** sends radioactive material through the blood stream, measuring how the brain and tissue are working, and detecting brain tissue disease.
- **DIT: Diffusion Tensor Image** may be effective in registering brain damage because it images the flow of water and is able to image the direction of water flow in the brain.

Unless there is a mass growth, bleeding or a cracked skull, most medical tests will not tell you of a brain injury. For example, the CT and MRI cannot tell the difference between a damaged brain and a healthy brain.

Concussion Recovery

The Stages of Recovery

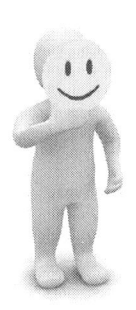

I had a client who was a highly visible professional athlete. She was a go-getter who could conquer the world. Then she suffered a severe concussion.

Frustrated, she wanted to know the ABC's of recovery in order to be healed by Tuesday at 6:00 pm. When I explained to her that a brain injury takes its own time to heal, she became very annoyed. She had pushed through every other injury and wanted to treat her head injury the same way.

I designed a routine and encouraged her to spend the summer at her family's cottage. There were few distractions, no overdosing on electronic gadgets or television. It was the ideal setting for recovery. She thought that she should do more. Instead of surrendering to the process and thriving on the little steps of recovery, she became anxious and impatient. This passionate drive became her biggest pitfall.

She did not understand that the healing process for a concussion is not a linear progression. It is an integrated spiral of stages that we go through, sometimes over and over.

Concussion Recovery

We must be assertive and determined in our healing journey. Aggressively pushing recovery is detrimental. Remember, slow and steady wins the race.

We must listen to our intuition and let our healing happen, painful step by joyous step.

These are stages as I see them:

1. **Denial and Confusion** "*There is nothing wrong with me. It is mind over matter.*"

    The reality of the injury might be ignored to avoid dealing with the concussion. This may last for weeks.

2. **Desperation and Shock** "*Oh no, I'm in trouble!*"

    We might snap unnecessarily at the people we care for. Our lives are breaking down. The accident might get replayed over and over in order for us to try to make sense of it. Mind chatter begins.

3. **FOG** - We are viewing the world through sheer curtains. Life stands still.

    Nothing seems real. The person might isolate themselves on purpose. There is no great emotion, just numbness.

4. **The Journey of the Return** - We start putting pieces back together.

    One day, we leave the fog. Much of life is still a concept. Like a spring flower breaking ground, life slowly becomes real again.

Concussion Recovery

5. **Uneasy Acceptance** *"Life is not as I recall."* — yes

    We find a way forward. Life is different. There is a mourning process of the loss of the person we once were and the skills we once had, as well as an appreciation of what we now have. — *I use to,*

    For example, I do not work in the same manner as before. — yes
    Sometimes I operate at a very advanced level of awareness. While, other times, compared to how I used to do things, I am the equivalent of a blind person walking on a tight rope across the Grand Canyon. — *Some what.*

    If someone met me for the first time, they would not know about my journey or my loss, and those who knew me before the accident do not understand that I am not the high functioning machine I once was. *Correct* — yes
    All the world's a stage
    Through the recovery process, our intuition will become highly developed if we let it. Listen and trust.

    No.

    Do you recognize yourself in any of these stages of recovery?

    Yes

Concussion Recovery

Different Kinds of Recovery

Like many other diseases, there are people who like to use the 'brain injured' label.

- There are those people who use their injury as an excuse to check out of life. *No!*

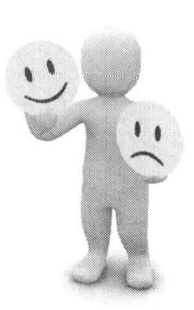

  I'm brain injured therefore all my behaviors are excusable. **No**

- There are those people who try to avoid worrying others.

  Don't worry about me. I have it all under control. **Yes**

- There is the group that hides in their closet, suffering in private. **Yes**

  No really. I am okay. — **Yes**

- There are those people who will break the rules against all odds and push the envelopes of the healing of their brain.

  I have no time for this. — **No**   *somewhat*

- There are those people who follow their intuition, honor their recovery time and rebuild their brains with positive thoughts and patience. **Yes** — *patience a challenge*

  I am rebuilding my brain with love and support. — **Yes**

  → *Jan me*

Which group will you be in?

Parts of the Brain

The brain is our body's computer. The two halves of the brain, which are called *hemispheres*, divide the thinking tasks.

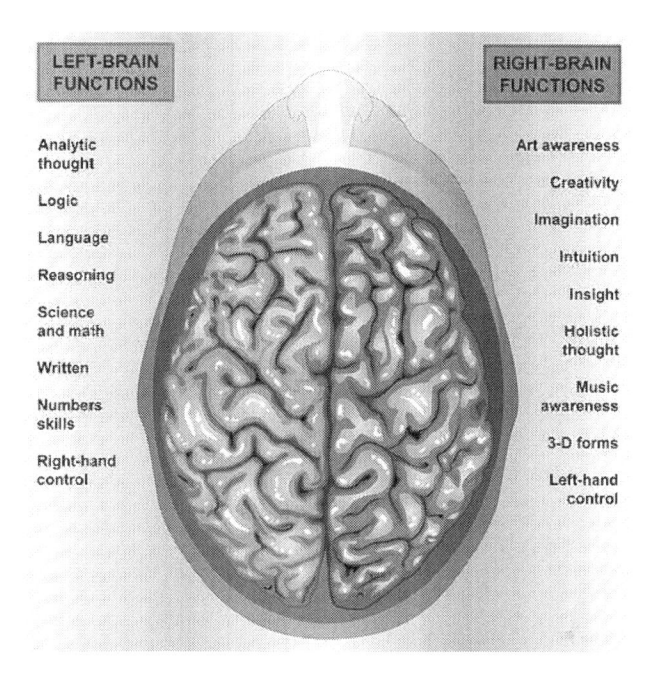

LEFT-BRAIN FUNCTIONS
- Analytic thought
- Logic
- Language
- Reasoning
- Science and math
- Written
- Numbers skills
- Right-hand control

RIGHT-BRAIN FUNCTIONS
- Art awareness
- Creativity
- Imagination
- Intuition
- Insight
- Holistic thought
- Music awareness
- 3-D forms
- Left-hand control

The left hemisphere is the side that deals with the human condition: math, factual & analytic processes, rational thought and objectivity. Responsible for the para-sympathetic nervous systems, it is our scheduler and our time manager.

The right hemisphere of the brain is the conductor of our creativity. It has no sense of time. Music, imagination, humor, dreams, poetry, architecture, drawing, and design are under the umbrella of the right brain. It is responsible for the sympathetic nervous system, which tells us to fight or flight in the face of too much stress.

Concussion Recovery

The right hemisphere controls actions on the left side of the body and the left hemisphere controls actions on the right side.

Is this getting a little complicated? You bet! Think of this:

- Our brain weighs only 3 pounds and has the consistency of gelatin.
- There are 100 billion cells called neurons in our brains.
- There are as many neurons as there are stars in the Milky Way.
- 100 brain cells can fit on the end of a pin.
- Each brain cell is equivalent to one computer.

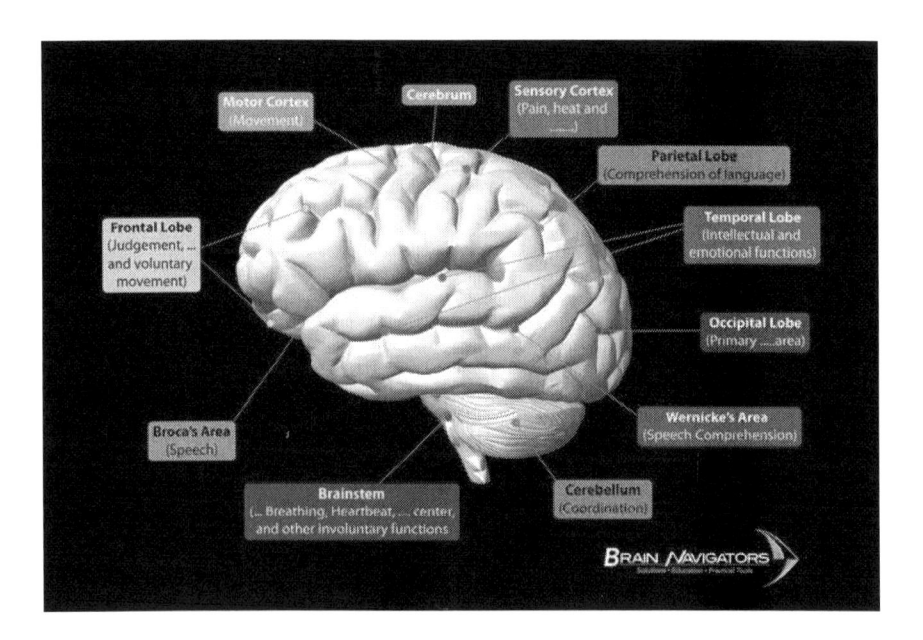

Diagram of the brain with labels: Motor Cortex (Movement), Cerebrum, Sensory Cortex (Pain, heat and ...), Parietal Lobe (Comprehension of language), Frontal Lobe (Judgement, ... and voluntary movement), Temporal Lobe (Intellectual and emotional functions), Occipital Lobe (Primary ... area), Broca's Area (Speech), Wernicke's Area (Speech Comprehension), Brainstem (... Breathing, Heartbeat, ... center, and other involuntary functions), Cerebellum (Coordination). Brain Navigators logo.

Cortex

The biggest part of the brain is called the *cortex* and it is further divided into four specialized areas called *lobes*.

The frontal lobe sits behind the forehead. It is responsible for organizing thoughts, and for helping to keep our behavior appropriate and attentive. If the frontal lobe is injured the possible results are:

- Loss of inhibitions
- Impaired mental flexibility
- Difficulty to prioritize tasks
- Lower motivation

The motor cortex is set behind the frontal cortex. It is approximately the size of your baby finger. It tells your body how to move its eyelid, wiggle its toes, lift an arm, etc.

The Broca is located in the frontal lobe. It is responsible for written and spoken language. If damaged, a person might show signs of *Broca's aphasia,* also called *expressive aphasia, motor aphasia,* or *non-fluent aphasia*. This means that:

- They have difficulty finding the words.
- They are not able to create complex sentences or understand language.
- Speech is telegraphic. Spoken sentences are short with only key words.
- Individuals have difficulty finding the correct word. Yet they are usually aware that their speech is improper. Example:

Concussion Recovery

"Two...ah, doctors ...and ah...thirty minutes. Two doctors...and ah...teeth. Yeah,"

sss tutter [handwritten]

Median section of the brain

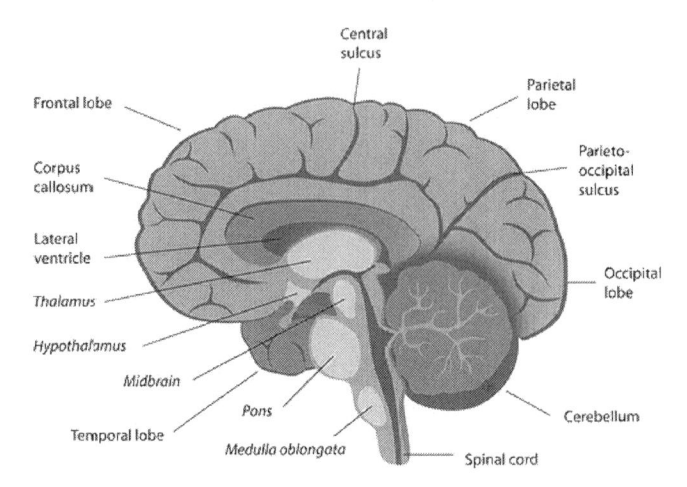

[Diagram of median section of the brain with labels: Frontal lobe, Corpus callosum, Lateral ventricle, Thalamus, Hypothalamus, Midbrain, Pons, Temporal lobe, Medulla oblongata, Central sulcus, Parietal lobe, Parieto-occipital sulcus, Occipital lobe, Cerebellum, Spinal cord]

The temporal lobe is beneath the ears. It is responsible for memory and hearing. This is where the brain learns new information and stores it to use later. If injured, possible results include: *? Damage above ear* [handwritten]

- Impairment or loss of long-term memory and language skills
- Difficulty placing words or pictures into categories
- Damage to the right causes the inability to recall non-verbal material, such as a drawing and music or loss of inhibition when talking.

Concussion Recovery

- Damage to the left impairs the ability to recognize words and can result in impaired memory for verbal material and in identifying smells.

Wernicke's Area is in the left temporal lobe. It makes sure that we form coherent sentences and that we understand the speech of others. If this specific area is injured:

- A person may lose the ability to understand spoken language, and read or speak with meaning.
- The injured person is often unaware of their problem and speaks in fluent, nonsensical babble. This is called 'Wernicke's aphasia'. For example: *"Anyway, this one here, and that, and that's it. This is getting in here and that's the getting around here, and that's it. This one and one with this one. And this one, and that's it, isn't it?"*

The parietal lobe is responsible to 'pull it all together' because it organizes the sensations. It is located above the temporal lobe and towards the back of the brain. If we see something or taste something, for example, the parietal lobe perceives and interprets the information. Possible results of injury to this part of the brain can cause:

- Apraxia: the inability to perform a specific movement. (Muscles are intact and able to perform that task under different circumstances.) For example, the patient is unable to touch their nose on command, but is able to scratch their nose.

Concussion Recovery

- Agnosia: the inability to recognize an object using a specific sense, even though that sense is basically intact. For example, the patient is unable to recognize an orange by sight, but can identify it by touch or smell.
- Other possible side effects are *Alexia* (word blindness), or *Agraphia* (writing impairment) and possible impairment to the ability to dress, wash, make or draw things. The person may neglect the opposite side of their body, even to the point of not recognizing their own limbs.

Within the parietal lobe, is the sensory cortex, which takes part in any feeling activity; any messages from a sense organ (like the eyes, nose, tongue, or ears) or messages of touch and temperature.

The occipital lobe is a bump that extends to the very back of the skull. It makes sense of the visual information that we receive.

- Damage to the right side results in loss of the left visual field of both eyes, while damage to the left results in loss to the right visual field of both eyes.
- Damage to both the left and right sides of occipital lobe can result in blindness, even though the eyes may be functioning normally. This is called cortical blindness.
- Damage to the front of the lobe means a difficulty in recognizing and interpreting familiar objects and faces.

Cerebellum

Located at the base of the brain, the cerebellum contains at least one-half of the brain's neurons, even though it is only 10 percent of the volume. Because it receives input from other parts of the brain and spinal cord, it controls the position and movement of our limbs and joints for balance and precise coordination.

Possible results of injury:

- Gait: standing or walking is not normal.
- Ataxia: unsteadiness or lack of coordination of the limbs, posture and gait.
- Tremor: parts of the body tremble uncontrollably. *Always*
- Hypotania: decreased muscle tone.
- Nystagmus: twitching of the eye.

Septal (Corpus Collosum)

With more than 300 million axons, the Corpus Collosum is the largest fiber bundle in the human brain. It sits between the cerebral hemispheres and ensures that each hemisphere has access to data from the opposite side of the body and surrounding environment. It is the brain's switchboard.

- Damage to the front of the corpus collosum can result in defective memory.

Concussion Recovery

- Damage to the rear can cause changes in behaviour and impaired judgment.

Side effects of an injury are as numerous as the functions of the brain.

According to Dana foundation, head trauma can manifest as:

- Depression
- Addiction
- Alcohol abuse
- Alzheimer's
- Panic disorders
- Autism
- Epilepsy
- Sleep disorders
- Headaches
- Parkinson's
- Tourette's
- Eating disorders
- Drug abuse
- Schizophrenia
- Cerebral palsy
- Stroke
- Muscular Dystrophy
- Shingles
- Learning Disabilities
- Pain
- Anxiety disorder
- ALS
- Obesity
- Financial problems
- Poor judgment
- Failed relationships
- Behavioral issues

Body Structure

No man is an island, nor is a brain injury an isolated island within our body.

The brain is our controller. Yet it depends on the rest of the body to transport information, especially through the spinal cord and around the spine. The messages pass through the narrowest part of our body - our neck!

If our posture is not aligned and this passage is not clear, nutrients do not flow through the brain and messages are not transported back and forth. Without fluid reaching the brain, it will wither and die.

For me, the emotions and pain were intense. My chiropractor worked wonders to align my spine. I also used hot yoga as a less aggressive way to achieve alignment. Do some investigation for yourself. Exercises to maintain alignment are perhaps the starting blocks in the race to recover.

Once again, you are the conductor of your body. Listen to it, learn from it and let your voice be heard.

You are healing your body from the inside. The professionals are looking at you from the outside. They can only work with the information you relate to them.

Concussions are serious and need to be treated seriously. If a head injury is not properly attended to, or if recovery is hurried, a blow to the head can lead to long-term damage. The affects may be very subtle and may not show up for years.

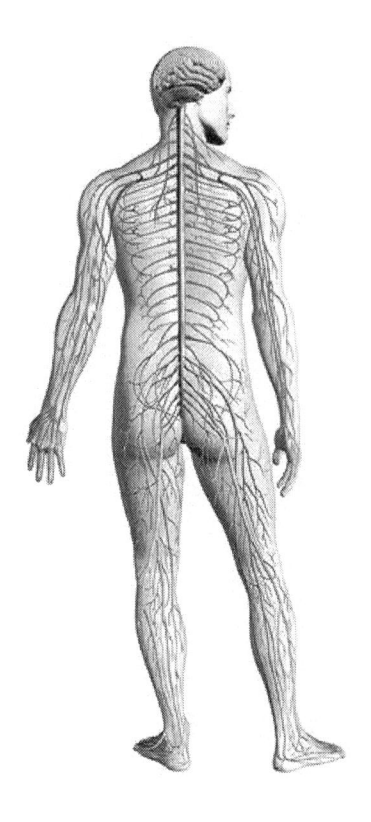

How complicated is our brain?

It is the most complicated arrangement of matter in the known universe.

Our brain has 100 billion nerve cells with 100 trillion connections.[iii]

Nutrition

Why is nutrition one of the first things that we work on?

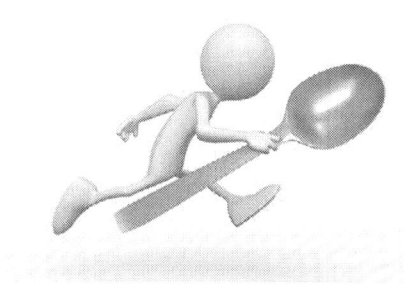

Simply put, your brain is bruised and needs some tender loving care. In order to repair the damaged area, your brain requires extra nutrients. A head injury is like a bomb that has just exploded in your head. All of the pieces are there. However, we need to find new ways to put the pieces together.

Being damaged, the brain must work much harder in order to complete simple tasks and to repair itself. Without proper nourishment, the cells cannot reconnect and heal. If necessary, your brain will take nutrients from other parts of your body, draining your adrenal glands and weakening your entire system. An injury to the brain changes the way our brains and bodies function and produce chemicals.

The human brain is only 2 percent of our total body weight. Yet, it needs roughly 20 percent of the total calorie intake in order to function correctly. If we do not consume good nutrients, the brain will rob other parts of the body. Other body systems will experience increased stress and possibly, disease in our bones, joints and muscles. So, right now, more than ever, you need to eat healthy food. — *No appetite*

Concussion Recovery

[handwritten: Yes. Janine helps ensure of it]

And what is healthy food? Healthy food is fresh, simple and minimally processed. Think about this: In a study of one million students in New York, those who ate lunches that did not contain additives, such as artificial flavors, preservatives and dyes, performed 14 percent better during IQ tests![iv] Clearly, your brain needs good fuel in order to function at its optimal level.

When you make a meal, serve in these proportions: One-quarter carbohydrates (pasta, rice, potato, grains); one-quarter protein (meat, eggs, fish, poultry, cheese); and one-half vegetables.

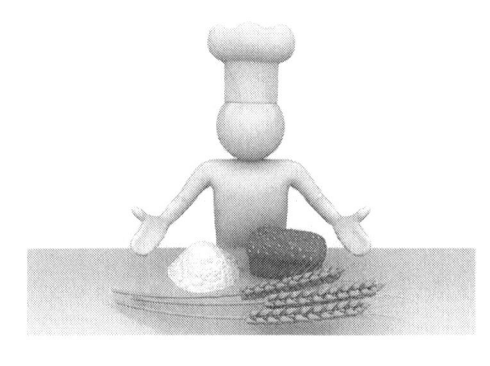

Buy the richest, most brightly colored vegetables and, at mealtime, try to see how colorful you can make your plate. Without realizing it, you will be offering your body a good dose of antioxidants. Put a rainbow of color on your plate. The antioxidants will help to pick up your energy.

Top 10 Brain Foods

Certain 'brain foods' boost the overall growth of your brain and improve your memory and concentration.

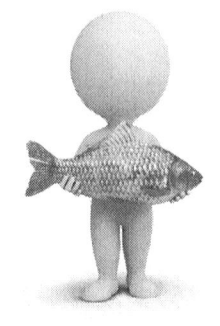

Concussion Recovery

#1: Salmon/Tuna/Mackerel

- Fish, which is rich in fatty acids, is an excellent source of Omega 3, fatty acids, DHA and EPA, which are all essential for brain growth and function.
- Research shows that people who eat salmon at least twice a week have sharper minds. Mental skills tests are a breeze for them.

#2: Eggs

- Eggs are always readily available and are a great protein source.
- Yolks also contain choline, which is absolutely necessary for brain function.

#3: Peanut Butter

- Both peanuts and peanut butter are excellent sources of thiamine which helps the brain and nervous system convert glucose into energy.
- Peanuts contain vitamin E, an antioxidant, which protects nerve membranes.

#4: Whole Grains — *Not so much*

- Whole grains are best because the fiber helps regulate the release of glucose and makes them slower to metabolize. Whole grains give a sustained level of energy as they do not turn to sugar as fast as white bread.

- Vitamin B in whole grains help build a healthy nervous system.

#5: Oats/Oatmeal

- Oats are 'grain for the brain.'
- Fiber-rich oats keep you energized throughout the morning by releasing their energy slowly.
- Oats are also rich in vitamins B, E, potassium and zinc, which help the brain and body to function at optimum levels.

#6: Berries

- Berries, such as strawberries, blueberries, acai berries and cherries contain powerful antioxidants.
- The richer the color intensity of a berry, the more nutritive value it has.
- Vitamin C is also present in berries, which is thought to prevent cancer.
- Those who consume berries regularly notice an improvement in their memory.
- The seeds of berries contain Omega 3 fatty acids.

#7: Beans

- Beans are an excellent brain food because they improve thinking by keeping the energy levels up.

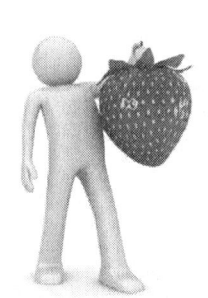

#8: Colorful Veggies

- Brightly colored, fresh vegetables are high in antioxidants, along with essential vitamins and minerals.
- Antioxidants boost immunity in addition to keeping the brain cells strong.
- Vitamins and minerals in vegetables help the body to function.

#9: Milk and Yoghurt

- The protein and B vitamins in dairy foods are essential for the growth of brain tissue and neurotransmitters.
- Milk and yoghurt are packed with protein and carbohydrates, which are sources of energy for the brain.

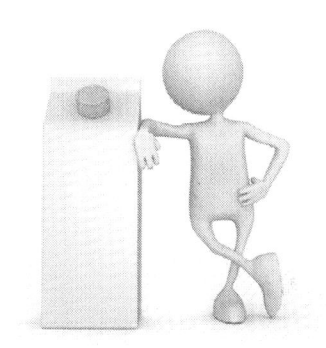

#10: Lean Beef, Oysters

- Lean beef and oysters are some of the best absorbed sources of iron.
- Iron helps with concentration and is especially important for growth.

Concussion Recovery

- Beef contains zinc, which aids memory.
- Vegetarians can use soy and black beans as alternatives to lean beef.

Food choices:

Consider these thoughts:
- If it's white, don't bite.
- Keep sugar intake to a minimum by reading labels. Natural sugars are the only sugars needed.
- After a very stressful day, cut down on carbohydrates (bread, potatoes, and baked goods) as they turn into sugar much faster. Try salad or vegetables with meat, poultry or fish.
- Foggy brain? Eat protein.
- Cut out or reduce unhealthy fats, deep fried foods and sodium.
- Steam or sauté, instead of deep-frying.
- Don't feel like cooking? Roast vegetables for one meal and serve for two.
- Soups and stews are great ways of increasing your vegetable intake during winter.
- Pineapples and papayas are very good for digestion.
- Avocados are good brain food.
- Substitute spinach for salad greens.
- Red and orange foods are high in antioxidants.
- Asparagus helps to clear the kidneys and bladder.

Concussion Recovery

Snacks:

Every few hours, try to eat a small healthy snack to keep the digestive system working and to regulate blood sugar. A few raw nuts, some cheese and fruit are fine. You may want to try juicing, as it is the fastest way to get minerals and vitamins into your body.

Breakfast:

The brain produces biochemical messengers, called neurotransmitters, which make connections. Without proper nutrients, neurotransmitters do not operate effectively. The more balanced the breakfast, the better the brain functions.

In addition, there are two types of proteins that affect neurotransmitters. Neuro-stimulants, such as the proteins that contain tyrosine, affect the alertness transmitters. Calming proteins such as dopamine and norepinephrine contain tryptophan to relax the brain.

The ideal breakfast contains complex carbohydrates and protein, with the right balance of both stimulating and calming foods.

A good breakfast starts your day right. Your brain is primed to learn and your emotions are prepared to behave.

Think grains, plus protein, plus fruit

- Scrambled eggs, toast, orange juice
- French toast topped with fruit or ham, orange juice or milk

- Cheese melted on toast with a piece of fruit
- Sausage in a bun with cheese, fruit
- Peanut butter and banana slices on brown toast, milk
- For a breakfast-on-the-run, try a smoothie with added minerals and protein.

Although our brain is the conductor and the motherboard of our bodies, we give little thought to growing and enhancing our brains.

We buy sunscreen or fancy creams to keep us youthful. However, we seldom think about giving the brain the right tools to work effectively. In addition, nutrition for the brain is often neglected because the results from the watering or nourishing of our brain are not immediately seen.

We need to feed our body premium foods for maximum performance. We must pump up the nutrition in our bodies.

Our brains depend on it.

Nutritional Supplements

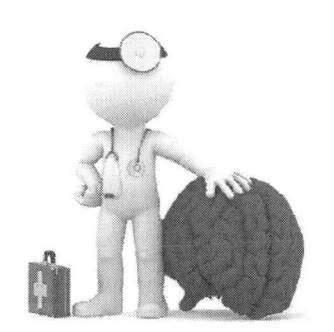

Sometimes our diet alone cannot provide sufficient nutrition. Our brains need super octane fuel right now. The vitamins and minerals in our food are not as plentiful as they once were. Simply put, we need supplements to pump up the nourishment in our bodies.

Our brain is like a garden. If you do not have good soil, the seeds you plant will just sit and stagnate. But seeds that are planted in good soil, with a little water and some warmth from the sun, will flourish in the nurturing environment.

Growing a garden is exactly the same as rebuilding your brain. With good nutrients, water and a few extra vitamins and minerals, our injured brains will flourish once again.

You might want to consider: ~~Always~~

Most importantly, drink water.

Our brains are made up of 70-80 percent water. Without water, our brains whither up. The messages cannot flow through the cells and the neurons of the brain. To keep our circulation clean, flush toxins from our body and ensure that our neurons can fire effectively, we must drink water.

Concussion Recovery

Always carry a water bottle with you and take small sips throughout the day. If you drink a litre of water at one time, it is like pouring a gallon of water over a plant. That large amount of water will flush out the kidneys and liver, washing away all of the nutrients in your body.

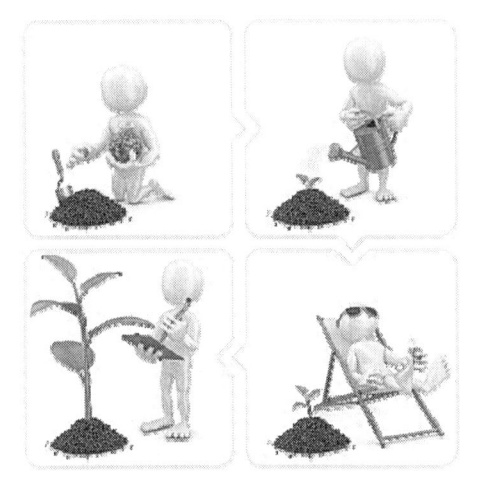

Drink at least 2 liters of water per day. As a general guide, for two pounds of body weight, an ounce of water is required. This means for every 1 kg, you need approximately 0.033 liters of water.

Coffee, pop, black tea, and liquor do not hydrate your body. They actually dehydrate you. To counteract the effects of each cup of dehydrating beverage that you consume, you will need to drink 3 cups of water, in addition to your regular amount.

Drink your water without ice. Water at room temperature is absorbed more easily than cold water. Cold water removes the precious energy that is needed for recovery, whereas warm water supplies it. One supports recovery, while the other sabotages it.

Drink coconut water. The high potassium content and antioxidants in coconut water make it more effective than commercial sport drinks.

Omega oils and Vitamin B

Scientists tell us that the brain is the fattiest organ in the body. Our brain is 90 percent fat. To nurture our brain and allow for easier blood flow, we must increase our healthy oil intake.

Remember when you have a brain injury, it is like you are stuck in traffic and need to take another route. More time and energy are needed to get to your destination.

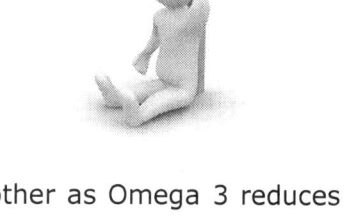

Remember, Omega 3 and 6 are required to be in balance with each other as Omega 3 reduces the damaging effects of Omega 6.

Omega 6 is found in eggs, poultry, cereals, vegetables and fish oils. It keeps our skin healthy and helps our blood to clot.

As with all things, some are better than others. Try to obtain the best quality Omegas possible. Each Omega will work on a different area of the brain.

You may be anxious, and even exhausted, from your efforts. Vitamin B is well known to help lift energy and keep depression at bay. A local health food store will recommend a Vitamin B supplement and possibly a good stress reducer to relax and calm your brain.

Anxious? Is your anxiety running high? Try a few Rescue Remedy® drops. Found at health food stores, they will help bridge the gap.

Astaxanthin

Astaxanthin *(pronounced asta-ZAN-thin)* increases strength and endurance and is one of the most powerful anti-inflammatory and antioxidant nutrients in the world. It is like the B Vitamins. It can cross the blood-brain barrier in order to protect the brain and nervous system, reaching into every part of the cell.

Seabuckthorn

Seabuckthorn is another powerful antioxidant, which contains considerable amounts of Vitamin C, E, A, as well as carotenoids. It is the only plant in the world that is known to contain betaine, folate, amino acids and Omega 3, 6, 7, and 9.

Thinking and feeling nutrients ... Vitamin B's

- At least 10 groups of B Vitamins work together to nourish the nervous system. They communicate between nerve cells to speed and even form neurotransmitters.
- A shortage of B1 can lead to psychosis and lower intelligence.
- B2 can help migraines, headaches and schizophrenia.

- B5 is the anti-stress vitamin. It controls adrenalin and boosts memory.
- B vitamins are thought to lower levels of homocysteine, a blood protein that is linked to heart disease, Alzheimer's and dementia.
- B-12 helps to form the myelin sheath that insulates nerves, boosts memory and reduces Alzheimer's.
- Folic acid helps prevent Alzheimer's. It deals with fatty acids in the brain.
- Older people may not be able to effectively absorb Vitamin B-12 because the ability to absorb folic acid diminishes with age. In addition to supplement, older folks may want to increase their consumption of vitamin-rich bananas, oranges, lemons, green leafy vegetables and lentils.
- B-12 is found in eggs, fish and meat (especially pork and offal).

Sources of B Vitamins

- B1 (thiamine): pork, whole grains and enriched grain products, such as bread, pasta, fortified cereals.
- B2 (riboflavin): organ meats, nuts, cheese, eggs, milk, lean meat, green leafy vegetables, fish, legumes, whole grains and yoghurt.

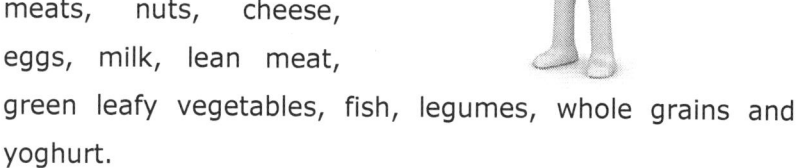

- B5 (panthothenic acid): meat, poultry, fish, whole grain cereals, legumes, vegetables and fruit.
- B6 (pyridoxine): chicken, fish, pork, liver, kidneys, nuts and legumes.
- B12 (cyanocobalamin): eggs, meat, fish and poultry.
- Folic Acid: green leafy vegetables, bananas, oranges, lemons, cantaloupes, strawberries and lentils.

Minerals

Minerals are the key leaders of the recovery team and are essential to recovering from a head injury. For example, magnesium is the conductor of all minerals. With low magnesium, the other minerals cannot work. Without sodium, other parts of the brain do not function properly. So, really, it is a balancing act. A high quality mineral supplement with trace minerals is recommended to provide the best nutrients for recovery.

Lack of minerals in the diet could be at the core of poor sleep patterns. Lack of sleep puts stress on the brain that, in turn, puts stress on the body.

Melatonin is a hormone that is produced in our brains. Stress can hamper its production so a supplement might be appropriate until balance is restored.

Minerals for Brain Power

- Calcium: strengthens bones and plays a vital part in nerve-signal transmission, as do potassium and sodium.

Concussion Recovery

- Potassium: balances sodium.
- Zinc, magnesium, copper and selenium: important for proper brain function.

Sources of minerals

- Magnesium: whole grains, legumes, nuts, sesame seeds, dried figs
- Potassium: apricots, avocados, bananas, melons, grapefruit, kiwi, oranges, strawberries, prunes, potatoes, pulses, meat, fish
- Calcium: fish with edible bones, sesame seeds, milk products
- Zinc: oysters, red meat, peanuts, sunflower seeds
- Selenium: meat, fish, Brazil nuts, avocados, lentils
- Manganese: nuts, cereals, brown rice, pulses
- Copper: offal, oysters, nuts, seeds, mushrooms, cocoa
- Sodium: meat, fish, dairy, eggs, smoked meats, pickles

Digestive Enzymes

When you have a brain injury, your ability to digest and absorb food is often severely affected. Scientists don't know why. A digestive enzyme that is taken with food will help digestion and decrease recovery time.

Weight gain

After a brain injury, most people gain weight. In the aftermath of an accident, the body creates more histamines and cortisol, which stress the adrenal glands and cause sluggish digestion.

Cortisol puts the weight on and the histamine causes nasal congestion.

HGH, hormonal growth hormone, is a controversial homeopathic product that helps bolster a sluggish metabolism and can counteract this stress on the adrenal glands.

If you are uncomfortable or have gained more than 20 percent of your body weight, you might want to see your doctor for help.

Still, your primary focus at this point must be to give the brain what it needs. Maybe your brain needs the fat in order to recover. Weight can always come off. You do not need to beat yourself up as a result of your increase in weight.

Hawaiian Spirulina

A nutritional algae, called Hawaiian Spirulina, is the world's purest most digestible natural source of concentrated protein, which yields immediate yet sustained energy. It helps detoxify the body by binding to toxins and eliminating them from the system.

Chlorophyll

Chlorophyll has the power to regenerate our bodies at the molecular and cellular level. It is known to fight infection, heal wounds and promote the health of the circulatory, digestive, immune and detoxification systems. Chlorophyll consumption increases the number of red blood cells and, therefore, increases oxygen utilization by the body.

Royal Jelly

Royal Jelly, which is made by bees, is the only natural source of pure acetylcholine. It has antibacterial and antimicrobial properties. Royal Jelly helps with mental conditions and is well known for its rejuvenating properties.

Herbs

The healing powers of herbs have been forgotten by modern medicine yet their strength remains. Consult with an herbalist for a blend that is right for you.

Feeling sluggish? Green foods, such as kelp, chlorella, alfalfa and wheat grass are also effective chelators or natural cleansers.

Memory deficency? Why not try gotu kola, Siberian ginseng, ginkgo biloba, wild oats, peppermint or rosemary?

Anger, frustration, anxiety, or depression giving you a problem? Try kava kava, St. Johnswort, passionflower, gotu kola, schezandra, Siberian ginseng, wild oats, stinging nettle, calamun root or prickly ash bark.

In quick summary, these supplements are highly recommended additions to your diet:

- Water: approximately 2 liters/day for better connections between neurons
- Mineral supplements for better communication between the cells and neurons of your brain
- Omega oils, fish oils
- Chlorophyll, Royal Jelly, Spirulina, Astaxanthin, Seabuckthorn
- Vitamin B for help with our thinking and feeling capacity
- Digestive Enzymes for nutrient absorption

Remember that you are the Cadillac of vehicles, not a pedal car. Get the best quality supplements and vitamins that you can.

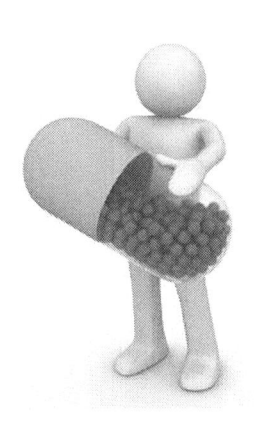

Sleep

There were days when I was asleep more than I was awake. I felt like a 100 year spell had been cast over me. Yet, I just couldn't sleep. When my doctor diagnosed me as depressed, I was so bewildered. My sleep patterns were all over the board. I was in physical discomfort from the accident and I was trapped in a roller coaster ride of feelings. I knew there was something wrong with me. But I didn't think I was depressed.

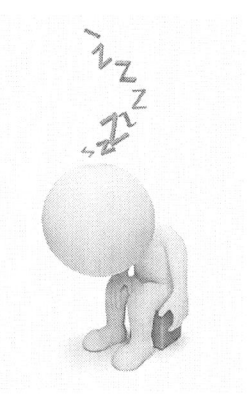

Then, I realized that I need to sleep when my brain is overloaded. But I never got a deep sleep. There are many things you can try. Remember that head injuries are as different from each other as people are.

Drugs

Drugs will not remove the demons that you will need to control. There is a risk of grogginess the next day or even of developing an addiction. At the onset of your injury, drugs may be needed to stop swelling, bleeding or pain. But they should not become a crutch.

Night time routine

Your conscious and subconscious paint the pictures on the canvas of your brain at night. So let your thoughts and

Concussion Recovery

experiences be happy ones. Your bruised and torn brain requires a little extra care in order to reshape your canvas.

Be consistent in your routine. If possible, do not exercise in the evening because it may keep you awake. Wind down slowly.

For a couple of hours before bedtime, surround yourself with things that are pleasant and joyful. Listen to happy music, watch a funny movie. Let your mind relax in joy.

The news, horror movies, violence and death, or music containing depressing messages, will all contribute to the creation of our world. With a bruised brain, we are more vulnerable to negative or strange thoughts.

To minimize mind chatter, let the subconscious know clearly what you want. Sometimes, while lying in bed, I tell my mind, *"I am going to sleep for x hours. I am going to wake up 100 percent rested."* Then, I repeat this. Tap touching techniques (which are explained later on) are also good activities for clearing the mind in preparation for a proper sleep.

When the entire world rests on your shoulders, write a list of all of the things that you are grateful for, and then read that list aloud. It is amazing when we stop our pity party, both our world and our attitudes change. The more positive we can be, the faster we can heal. There is always someone worse off than you. In reality, we all live a pretty privileged life in this part of the world.

Concussion Recovery

A prince or princess mask

You may go through a phase when you are so sensitive to light and noise that every little thing will disrupt your sleep. When you sleep with a mask over your eyes, you have added another tool to your toolbox that can allow you to awaken feeling peaceful and rested. *+ Ear plugs*

Aromatherapy *No*

We are very sensitive to smells. Lavender is a very soothing scent. Before bed, put some on your wrists or arms, or under your nose. It will encourage you to focus on deep breathing.

A Warm Bath *Do not like baths*

If you like, try a warm bath containing Epsom salts (1-2 cups) and a few drops of lavender. Epsom salts are magnesium sulphate, and magnesium is the conductor of all of the minerals in your body. Epsom salts help to produce serotonin, draw toxins from the body, sedate the nervous system, reduce swelling and relax muscles. In short, it is a win-win for everyone.

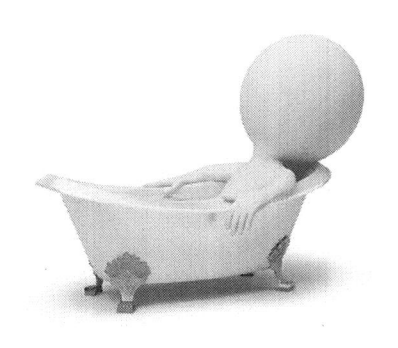

lots! [handwritten annotation with bracket pointing to headings]

Concussion Recovery

Bananas and Warm Milk

They say that imbalanced minerals are the main cause of sleeplessness. Bananas contain potassium and warm milk is full of calcium. So they are just right for a bedtime snack.

Melatonin

In the shake-up of a concussion, sometimes the brain stops producing the chemical, melatonin, which helps us to sleep. Until balance is achieved again, a melatonin supplement, which you can obtain from the health food store, will help you get to sleep easily. I did not have any side effects.

Breathing *Do this every night* [handwritten]

Breathing in for a count of 6, and then out for a count of 6 will shift energy and dissipate stress. Even before I had an Acquired Brain Injury ("ABI"), I always used to breathe in the good and breathe out the bad. I did not have to name the good or the bad. But it really helped when I was stressed. In reality, the exercise was clearing my subconscious. I also did not know about the variety of different types of breathing that exist. Nor did I realize that nearly every different style of breathing causes a different feeling.

Relaxation tapes

I had tapes of sound waves that my neurologist recommended but, for me, the results were minimal. Nature and yoga meditation tapes worked better. You might have do try various tapes until you find what is right for you.

Our thoughts

When we go to sleep, we should spend some time thinking happy, healthy thoughts. Think joy. Think of what brings you joy. Think of what makes you grateful. Then, ask for what you want. Yes, you could use the word *prayer*. Connect with whatever is your figure of strength, and then ask for help to heal your injuries. You can be as specific as you want here. The clearer and more precise your request is, the better.

If this is too much for you, try a different technique. When you are breathing, lie in stillness, breath silver or gold sparkles through your entire body. Allow the light to flow through the top of your head, through every part of your skull, brain, nose, throat, neck, spine, through your entire body, through any aches or pains, through to the arches in your feet, and then down to the center of the Earth. This will have a healing and calming effect on you.

When you wake in the middle of the night

There is a series of exercises, which were designed by Dorothy Espiau, which certainly allowed me to sleep. When these exercises are practiced throughout the day, our world definitely becomes a better place. Performing the series of exercises takes only about 2-3 minutes. Sleep then becomes easier and deeper.

Concussion Recovery

Cross touch at the hairline helps to stop the busy mind. Touching the top of the head helps to bring your attention to the present time. When I would awaken in the middle of the night for various reasons, I would do these exercises and quickly return to an incredible sleep.

Without a sound sleep, the brain cannot heal itself, and then it is extremely difficult to function the next day.

Naps

Naps mend the brain. Nap when you need it.

Shortly after the accident, my head would get so full that it felt like it might burst. My brain felt like my stomach did after eating a huge Christmas feast, when my eyes had been bigger than my stomach. The only cure for this tightness in my head was to nap, even for only 5 minutes.

If I was around traffic noise, fans, or crowds of people, my head would fill up very quickly. My full head was the dictator of both my actions and my body. So, even now, when I go into overload, I take a catnap. In a short amount of time, I can go from being overwhelmed to thinking, 'Okay, bring it on! I am ready.'

In summary

Do not be afraid to sleep. Sleep when and where you need to.

- For a good night's sleep, make your bedroom a peaceful dark sanctuary and make your routine as consistent as possible. ✓
- Do not feel guilty. — ? of being a dependent
- Think joy. — fluff
- Luxuriate in this time. Fuk right off. Ha!
- Healing and re-programming your brain takes time. It is not like training for a race or an exam. — Yes

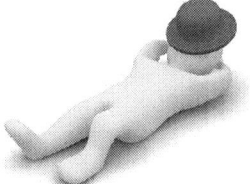

Listen to your body. It will not lie.

Body willing to train + excercise.

Operating on minimal calories, due to no appetite.. Low fuel = low energy

Concussion Recovery

Emotional Aspects

If you have ever been on a roller coaster, you will know that living life with a head injury or concussion is like riding the most horrific roller coaster in the world.

Again, let's be clear, all head injuries are different. The angle and the velocity of the hit determine the location and extent of the damage, as well as the individual's recovery time.

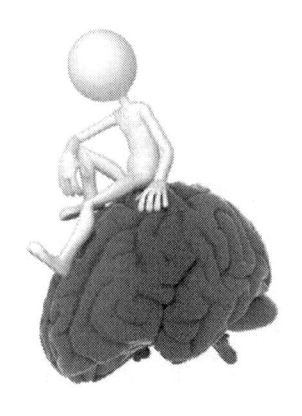

[handwritten: Have not fallen through cracks - good - support resource]

Having fallen through the cracks myself; I would say that, emotionally, the worst part is being told that you are perfectly fine by an authority figure, such as a doctor or psychiatrist, even though you know your thinking is off. *[handwritten: Yes! by some - most educated on TBI]*

If you share your wild thoughts, the doctor will pressure you to take medication to raise serotonin levels and cause further numbing. You might be classed as psychotic, delusional or whatever the trendy label of the hour is. Joining the drug numbing world will delay healing time by the same amount of time that the medication is taken. *[handwritten: Not pressured to take drugs]*

Most likely, the doctors helping you now did not know you and your abilities before the accident so you have an important role in understanding and diagnosing your injury.

Concussion Recovery

Of course, there are situations when medication may be required or recommended. Medication offers short term solutions and should not be the first line of defense.

Short term

Many healthier options await you on the road to recovery. They are not always easy.

Yes, some days, the voyage to the town of Sanity and Health may indeed be filled with difficult detours.

Stress

The greater the stress in your life, the more chaotic your brain will become and the harder it is function.

To reduce the emotional roller coaster in your mind: *Appetite?*

Eat the right nutrients to promote growth and healing.

Create peace in your physical surroundings.

- Reduce white noise: microwaves, cell phones, flashing signs, traffic, bathroom and kitchen fans, etc. Be very cognitive of white noise; it inhibits your brain's ability to repair itself.

- Reduce outside stimulants. Too much stimulation will crash and burn you faster than you can imagine. Even though you may enjoy it or be totally unaware of it, the stress will creep up on you. I used to work at my computer, answer the phone and listen to the radio all at the same time. But now I get tired very fast. Working in silence is best. *Yes*

Concussion Recovery

- During my recovery time, I had the great privilege of traveling the world with a friend. This was an incredible opportunity. However, all of the new sounds, smells, sights, lights and wonderful experiences that I did not want to miss simply put me in overload. I would crash. Sleep was my escape. After each trip, I would need to escape to the sanctuary of my home, which is both quiet and peaceful. No noise. No clutter. No people. Just solitude.

- Nature is a tremendously healing place, whether you choose to walk, work or play in it. Take time each day to be in nature. It will take your troubles away, grounding and revitalizing you.

Focus on YOU.

- Reduce the personal stress in your life, whether it is relationships or old emotional baggage that you have been carrying. Responsibilities in life need to be kept to a minimum.

- Make a list of your most basic responsibilities. Then go back and cut the list in half. This healing time is about YOU. You are learning to set new boundaries and take care of YOU.

- Do not feel guilty about taking this time for yourself. You are in the repair shop and your brain is getting an overhaul. Rebuilding your brain is a full-time job.

Concussion Recovery

Release the expectations of others.

- When someone looks at you, your brain injury will not be obvious to them. I remember when I had to attend court, I was nervous because my thinking was not clear. If I was put on the spot, I would 100 percent freeze, or worse, I would agree just to stop the situation. The judge said, "*Well you look fine, I'm sure you will do just fine.*" Inside, I was like a 5000-piece puzzle box. The pieces were all there. But the picture was not formed. Sometimes you need to explain yourself.

- You would get more empathy from a broken leg or a cut on your finger. People do not understand this silent invisible injury. Be patient.

Beware of addictions.

- Addictions are powerful, overwhelming and often a part of brain injuries. The brain is trying to reconnect. There is no easy way to deal with them. — *Beer? / beer — ? moderation?*

- Knowledge is power. Be aware of the risk of addiction and learn a new balance. — *Advised by Neuro's*

- Stay rested and healthy, with good nutrition, sleep and exercise. *Not realistic with current challenges. A goal.*

- Speak positive words to yourself. (Later in the workbook, I describe Brain Builders, which are very effective.) *Cluff*

Concussion Recovery

- To help speed along the healing process, remove the pressures and stress from your life.

Stay connected

- As a friend, I became forgetful and unreliable. I would repeat myself numerous times to the point of boredom, burst out with inappropriate comments or even forget what I had just said. One by one, piece by piece, my life and my friends were falling away. I had to make an effort to stay connected and explain myself.

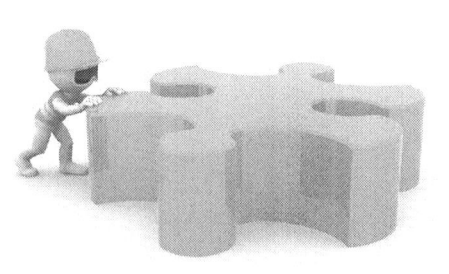

- Make sure that your need for solitude is balanced by positive social interaction. Isolation is debilitating. Yet, you do need time alone and the tranquility that solitude can bring.

- It helps if you have someone to advocate for you and to remind you of the progress you have made. However, be careful. Comparing your present self to your past self may set up too many expectations. *Jan the a advocate*

Create a refuge for yourself. Find little successes.

- During my escape times, I built a water feature in my yard. It was very healing and, at the end of the day, I would look at my accomplishments and feel good about myself. My yard was my saviour. *Nova.*

Concussion Recovery

The power of positive thought

Our thoughts create our world. When I have a 'pity party,' I attract negativity into my life. The spiral of depression and negativity can start taking over.

Positive thinking attracts the positive into our lives. The old saying, *'if you do not have something nice to say, do not say anything at all,'* is perhaps most pertinent for a person with a brain injury.

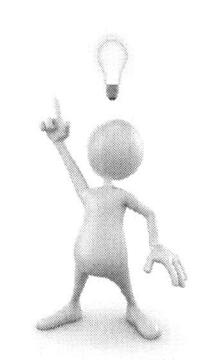

Learning the art of positive thinking is so important in retraining the brain and getting off the emotional roller coaster. If we can replace our negative thoughts with positive ones, we get on the road to recovery. *Am positive*

This method is the beginning of the new you that is taking control of your destiny. Henry Ford once said, *"If you think you can't you can't, if you think you can, you can."*

You can!

Getting the Upper Hand on Depression

There are 60-70,000 thoughts that go through our brain each day.[v] If even half of those thoughts are negative, the subconscious will pick up the negative thoughts at night and will play them over and over while we sleep. Then, we spiral down.

Concussion Recovery

We need to protect ourselves. Depression, addiction and suicide are some of the risks of brain injury. Our injury is misunderstood. Health professionals can let us down. We may feel shame and want to hide. The real issue is that the chemicals in our brains have been shaken up and they need time to settle.

Be aware of the spiral down. With a brain injury, old thought patterns and programs are replaced with new thoughts for the creation of a new person - a new happy person.

We must constantly invite our brains to release endorphins to stimulate our system. How much happiness can you tolerate? Try to raise your serotonin level.

Sometimes the depression moves like waves through the body. Listen. Know your triggers. Recognize that when you start to slide down, you need to change your activity. Do something that will make you happy.

To stay out of the downward cycle, surround yourself with positive people and positive experiences. Boost your serotonin levels with exercise. The fresh air flushes out negative thoughts and brings in fresh oxygen. But most importantly, be gentle with yourself.

Go to sleep on a happy note. Read and re-read the list of things for which you are grateful. Say 'No' to guilt, overexertion and problems that are not your own. Seek help if you need it. You are not alone.

Concussion Recovery

Think of this:

- With every heart beat, 20-40% of the blood goes to the brain
- Three full soda cans of blood flow through the brain every minute
- In that minute, the brain will absorb the oxygen from that blood
- `Life is good. Life is better. I like my life,' is an excellent Brain Builder.

Each person is unique, and so is the injury and recovery process. Here are a few other little tricks of imagination and visualization that you may want to try:

1. Take a few deep breaths in through your mouth and envision yourself pushing the breath out through your heart area. If you are unable to do this, take 6 deep breaths in and out for a count of 6. Now, with your eyes closed, imagine a halo that is about 4-6 inches wider than your head. This halo is resting on your shoulder. In your mind's eye, imagine the halo floating up to encircle your head at the level of your forehead. Breathe in the contentment that you feel. You have potential and you are a very capable person.

2. Our words form our worlds. They can lift us up or knock us down. So pay close attention to the words you use. The word, *can't* is about powerlessness and victimization. Erase it from your vocabulary! Your words resonate and

Concussion Recovery

continuously re-enforce your thoughts. If you say, "*I can't walk.*" Guess what? You won't be able to walk. Perhaps try using words like, "*I am learning to walk better, every day I am walking better, walking is becoming easier.*" Acknowledge what you are becoming. But do not wallow in your pity of can't.

3. When you really feel rotten, I recommend that you lie to yourself. Yes, that is true. Convince yourself that you are feeling well. You may have a chemical imbalance or you may be over-tired. Don't let your negative thoughts create a negative world for you. You have the power! Your situation is temporary. Be gentle and kind to yourself.

4. Focus on what you want. Create a memory board from magazines of everything that brings you joy. This is your visual 'cheat sheet.'

5. Force a smile on your face. Get dressed and visit someone older who does not receive many visitors. Feel the joy that you bring them.

6. If you feel lonely or sad, listen to music, watch a funny movie, dance, etc.

7. Get into a routine and connect with someone who can be a buddy to walk with, exercise with, attend social events with, etc. Agree that you will encourage each other to get up and go for a walk, even when you do not feel like it. Set a goal for both of you, such as losing inches or pounds. Make it a

Concussion Recovery

challenge that is fun for both of you. For example, whoever misses exercise buys the coffee.

8. Read the section on `Brain Builders` and try this one: *"I am happy. I am having fun. I have lots of friends. There is always someone around to call who appreciates me. I am a magnet for my positive desires."*

Mind Chatter

STOP is a wonderful word that can make a real difference if you use it in your self-talk. Just say, "Stop!"

For a more long-term solution, you might try another walking exercise:

1. Write these phrases down:
    - I choose an integrated mind.
    - I compute.
    - I choose to be single minded.
    - I feel single minded.
    - I am single minded.
    - I compute.
    - I choose an integrated mind.
    - I feel like I am integrated mind.
    - I have an integrated mind.
    - I choose to be whole minded.
    - I feel whole minded.
    - I am whole minded.

2. Go for a walk and repeat these phrases for a few minutes.
3. Enjoy your walk for a while, and then repeat the phrases again. If you can speak out loud, the sound of your own voice will resonate throughout your body and mind.

Our words are very important. They create our thoughts.

Brain Builders

A `Brain Builder` is the best way that you can take control of mind chatter. Think of your brain as a little child. It is up to you to nurture your brain and teach it how to speak, think, create, move and feel.

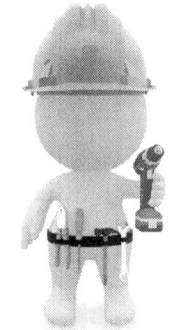

Start talking to your brain. Lay down the law. Tell your brain how it is going to behave and what thoughts are appropriate. Your conscious mind must direct your subconscious.

A Brain Builder is a step-by-step way to direct your recovery.

1. Make a list of all of the things that you are grateful for, and then bring it with you.
2. Start your Brain Builder by inhaling through your nose for a count of 6, and then exhaling forcefully through your mouth for a count of 6. Do this 6 times.
3. With your gratitude list in hand, go for a walk and repeat your Brain Builder. If you are somewhere private, speak out loud. This should take 10-15 minutes.

4. Take a few more breathes in and out, and then enjoy the beauty of your walk.
5. If you are still not feeling better when you return from your walk, repeat the phrases in your gratitude list for the last 5 minutes.

Sometimes you might want to use other statements, such as these:

- I choose to be happy. I feel happy. I am happy.
- I chose to have clear thinking. I feel like I have clear thinking. I am thinking clearly.
- The phrases, I choose, I feel and I am, are very powerful words that can be used alone as your Brain Builder.

This process takes time. Do not expect results to happen overnight. It takes 6 weeks to change a habit and we are changing your brain, which may not yet be working on all cylinders.

You are the conductor. You choose the music of the symphony that is playing in your head.

In Summary

A brain injured person lives in the 'feeling world' more than others do. We are much more likely to ask, *"How are you feeling?"* rather than *"What are you doing?"*

This awareness and joy in the present moment is a strength that we must cultivate. Take time to watch wasps as they build their nest. Notice how a bud slowly changes into a flower. We must build our capacity for delight in little things.

In this rerouting stage, the pitfalls of depression are so dangerous. Have your gratitude list ready. When you feel yourself slipping into these dark places, consciously talk to yourself. Repeat what you are grateful for and what you are going to be. You will get there.

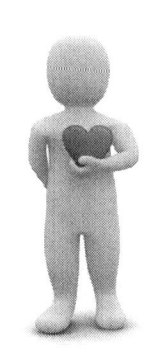

How do you eat an elephant?

One bite at a time.

Gently.

Post Traumatic Stress Disorder

Post Traumatic Stress Disorder (PTSD) is a reality of a brain injury. The event that caused your injury has been imprinted on your memory. Your whole body has experienced trauma. The impact might have exploded areas in your brain. Your body might be out of alignment.

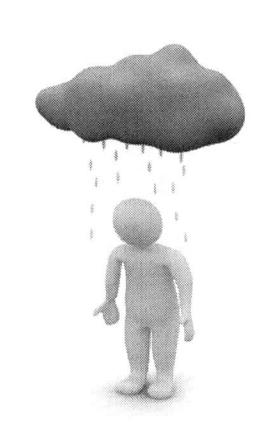

As painful as it may be, PTSD needs to be addressed and removed from your energy field. Otherwise, the stress of the situation will impede your healing. Time alone may not be enough to heal.

Diagnosing PTSD can be difficult because it comes in so many forms, such as nightmares, anxiety, sweats, etc.

The first step is to acknowledge yourself and your experience. Then, maintain a healthy lifestyle of good nutrition, sleep and exercise.

Finally, consider some specific treatment. I have tried each of these.

You are the judge of what works for you. Each injury is different. You are the leader of your return to health.

Visualization

Depending upon your situation and the trauma you are experiencing, you can either try this on your own or with a healing practitioner. In a very relaxed state, go back in tIme and relive the situation. However, just before the incident takes place, change the dynamics of the situation. Perhaps you left a little earlier, and then stopped and had a coffee with a friend.

With a mild case of PTSD, there are other simple techniques that may help, such as using the breathing techniques to relax, placing all of your nightmares of the event in a violet or pink balloon, and then letting them drift away. Or simply surround yourself with white light. Envisioning will change the dynamics of the injury and it is a really large part of the healing process.

Geo-Tran

Developed to remove insistent thought codes and to reprogram your energy field, Geo-Tran is a non-evasive treatment that is so simple that you will think that nothing is being done. Geo-Tran practitioners who are trained in this complicated technique can make positive changes to your stress and other negative symptoms.

EMDR

Eye Movement Desensitization Reprocessing can be effective. Be sure to find a practitioner that uses this technique manually. No machines! Your brain is repairing. Be gentle on yourself.

Tap touching

If you have problems with memory, you may find the steps in each exercise difficult to grasp. But trained practitioners and a few really good YouTube videos may be enough to help you learn this wonderful technique.

Hypnosis

Some people have had great results with hypnosis. You can listen to CDs or visit a trained professional hypnotist.

In Summary

When the trauma is removed from the energy field, the blocks to healing are also removed and there is less attraction to further head injuries. Health does return. The life you are experiencing now is temporary.

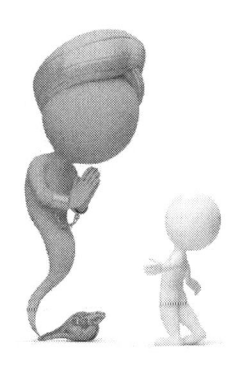

You are special and you were given a gift. You are just learning how to recognize and use it.

Physical Exercise

Physical exercise is so important for everybody in order to keep a healthy attitude and a strong body. But exercise is even more important in the rejuvenation of a bruised brain.

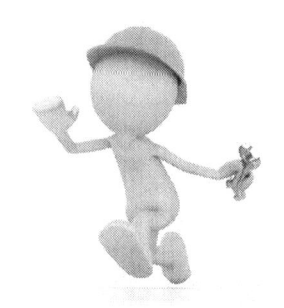

Prior to my accident, I swam, walked, ran and sweated through boot camp classes at least 3 days a week. My work was also very physical. I ran up and down hills, climbed under houses and unloaded truckloads of building supplies.

About a week after the accident, the curtains came down on me. I had been fine but when I returned home one day, feeling a little off and a little tired, I could not get out of my truck. Tears of pain flooded down my face. I needed to get changed in a hurry for an appointment but my body could not move. A good half hour passed before I reached the top of my steps.

The impact from the other vehicle had rearranged every structure within my body. I had the adult version of the 'shaken baby syndrome.'

This was really the death of the old me. Before the accident, I had no idea of the journey I would embark on. Yet here I am today, writing this book, having walked through the valley depths into the sun of recovery.

Concussion Recovery

These tools help:

Breathe

We can do a lot with our breath. Actually, deep breathing is a physical exercise.

If we are laying in a body cast, unable to move a muscle, the one exercise that is available to us is breathing.

Strangely, there is nothing easier than breathing. We have done it all of our lives. But conscious breathing takes some concentration and focus. There are so many different ways to breathe that I could write a whole book on breathing.

These exercises will focus on circulating more oxygen throughout our bodies in order to feed the most important muscle in our body - our brain.

- Breathe in through your nose for a count of 6, and then out for a count of 6. Do this 6 times, breathing out through your mouth, pushing the air completely out of your body.
- Breathe in through your nose for a count of 6, and then out for a count of 6. Do this 6 times, breathing out through your nose.
- Breathe in through your nose, for a count of 6, and then out for a count of 6. Do this 6 times, breathing out of the arches in your feet.
- Breathe in through your nose for a count of 6, and then out for a count of 6. Do this 6 times, breathing out into the area of the pain in your body.

Excellent! Now this takes a little imagination. Pretend that there is a tube that runs through your body, from the top of your head, through your brain, neck and spine, and then out through the bottom of your toes. The tube is very flexible and moves easily with your body.

- Breathe in through the imaginary tube that starts at the top of your head, for a count of 6, and then out for a count of 6. Do this 6 times, breathing out of your mouth.
- Breathe in through the imaginary tube that starts at the top of your head, for a count of 6, and then out for a count of 6. Do this 6 times, breathing out of your throat chakra.
- Breathe in through the imaginary tube that starts at the top of your head, for a count of 6, and then out for a count of 6. Do this 6 times, breathing out and down your spine.
- Breathe in through the imaginary tube that starts at the top of your head, for a count of 6, and then out for a count of 6. Do this 6 times, breathing out through the tips of your toes.

With our imagination flowing freely, let's try that last exercise with colors. We are going to bring colors through the body and let the vibration be felt. The power you possess inside you will work its magic.

Why color?

Color vibrates at different frequencies and we respond accordingly. Think of how you feel when you walk into a room that has been painted all black. How do you feel? Now

Concussion Recovery

imagine that you are walking into that same room, but that it has been painted yellow. Your feeling changes, doesn't it?

Restaurants are painted different colors in an attempt to dictate the length of time that you stay. Music is played according to the dinner hour. You walk into a fast food restaurant. How is it painted? How long do you stay? How do you feel? Then, you walk into a fine dining restaurant. What are the colors? How do they make you feel?

Yes, color heals all of the parts of your body that are in pain. A caregiver or guide could remind you of what has to be done. But this is really about you learning the power of you. These exercises stimulate the right side of your brain and get your creative mind working again.

I like to imagine the color gold. Gold is a warm soothing color to breathe through my body. White and sparkling sliver heal and melt away pain. This does take some time and patience to learn how to breathe out your pain spots. But it is well worth the effort.

I cannot stress enough that each head injury is different and that abilities to conquer any one exercise may prove to be a challenge. Remember that you are the conductor of your own brain. When it comes to learning a new task, you are simply teaching your symphony a new repertoire.

Give these breathing exercises a couple of tries with different colors to see if it works for you at this time.

- Breathe in white through the imaginary spot on the top of your head, for a count of 6, and then out for a count of 6. Do this 6 times, breathing out of your mouth.
- Breathe in white through the imaginary tube that starts at the top of your head, for a count of 6, and then out for a count of 6. Do this 6 times, breathing out of your throat chakra.
- Breathe in white through the imaginary tube that starts at the top of your head, for a count of 6, and then out for a count of 6. Do this 6 times, breathing out and down your spine.
- Breathe in white through the imaginary tube that starts at the top of your head, for a count of 6, and then out for a count of 6. Do this 6 times, breathing out through the tips of your toes.

Walking

Your next level of physical activity is most likely going to be walking. Do what you can when you can! Try to work up to 3 miles (4 kilometers) a day. The more you huff and puff during those first few walks, the more blood circulates through your brain. Remember to listen to your body though. Respect your own limits.

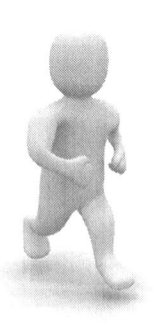

Exercise

Exercise stimulates the brain.

Although you may sometimes loath it, exercise releases endorphins that make you happy - even exhilarated. The advantage of the exercise is that it flushes the brain with a fresh flow of oxygen. Blood rushes through the runways of our brains and serotonin is released.

Different exercises work on different parts of the brain, in the same way that sit-ups work the stomach muscles, and push-ups work the arms and chest. Studies that have taken place of the brain have shown that different kinds of exercise will help to grow a healthy brain. We need to think of the brain as a muscle. To be healthy, the brain needs to be exercised, whether that is by playing a mental game or by performing physical exercise. For now, we are only going to deal with the physical exercise.

According to boot camp memory guru, Tony Buzan, we need to work on four areas of physical fitness in order to strengthen the brain:

1. Poise
2. Aerobic training and fitness
3. Flexibility
4. Strength

Concussion Recovery

Poise

Poise is the perfect balance of the body, in which all aspects of our muscles and skeletal systems are properly aligned. All of the body's signals run from the brain, through the neck and the spine. There are hundreds of thousands of signals that travel though this narrow part of the body. Yet, the neck and spine are often 'the forgotten soldiers' of our bodies. If this passage is not clear and our posture is not aligned, the messages cannot get back and forth to/from the brain. This includes getting food or fluid to the brain itself. If fluid does not reach the brain, it will wither and die.

Try lying on the floor with a heating pad on your neck and spine. When you feel warm, lie face down and simply turn your head so that your ear is resting on the floor. Let your big toes touch and let your feet flop open. Your arms should be at your sides with the palms turned up. Your thumbs should be close to your body. With the heating pad to loosen things up for you, hold this position for 3-5 minutes, and then change sides. If you are watching television, try this position during each commercial, first with the right ear on the floor, and then the left.

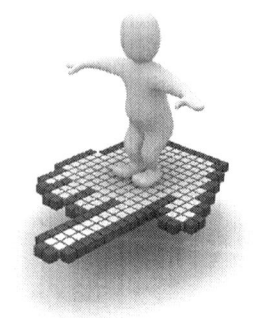

With good posture, blood flows through your body more easily. If you are sedentary, you are supplying less vital oxygen to your body and, particularly, to your recovering brain. This puts a strain on your entire body. Your blood is not circulating effectively and this slows down the transmission of 'Nerve Knowledge,' causing pain in the process.

Proper poise allows fluidity of movement and a natural flow of all of your mental and physical energies.

Exercise: Take a sip using the straw in front of you. Now crumple up the straw. Try taking a drink. Imagine your blood trying to push its way through the straw. The effort puts strain on your heart, lungs and blood vessels

Aerobic Exercise

Aerobic exercise is anything that creates a sweat, and stimulates the heart and lung activity. Fast walking, running, swimming, cycling and rowing are exercises, which will help to stimulate the brain. (Remember though to keep yourself hydrated with little sips of water throughout your workout and throughout your day.)

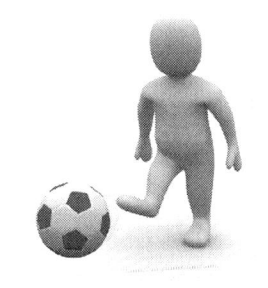

Aerobic exercise builds stamina and endurance, and forces the heart to pump more life-giving oxygen throughout the body. Studies have shown that, even just one-half hour of exercise, 3 times per week, improves blood circulation, increases

Concussion Recovery

brainpower and boosts memory. Imagine, regular exercisers score higher on IQ tests![vi]

Other studies show that aerobic exercise creates new capillaries and new neuron activity throughout the brain, within 3 days of performing the activity.[vii] This is encouraging because it shows that we can take control. We must not roll over and accept that the party is finished. We have a responsibility to get our brains working well again.

Remember, your brain takes up only 2-3 percent of your body weight and many of the capillaries that carry the blood to your brain are microscopically small. Yet, a whopping 20-40 percent of the blood goes directly into your brain, with every beat of your heart!

Other benefits of exercise include:

- You will have better quality sleep and you will need less sleep. — *No evidence yet*
- After your aerobic workout, your brain is better equipped to cope with stress and take in new information. *Yes*
- There is a correlation between physical and mental health. When your body is flexible, so is your mind. Creative ideas flow more easily.
- Exercise protects your internal organs.
- Exercise increases your confidence. You look good; you feel good. *Yes*
- Serotonin is naturally produced and released.
- Exercise stops the downward cycle of depression. *No*

Concussion Recovery

Aerobic exercise is important. How can you fit it into your schedule?

Flexibility *Yoga*

The flexibility of your body promotes the flexibility of your brain. Although there are many ways to increase your flexibility, I particularly like hot yoga! Unlike other types of exercise, the yoga room is hot and humid! The process detoxifies your body and transforms even the sorest body into a flexible elastic band.

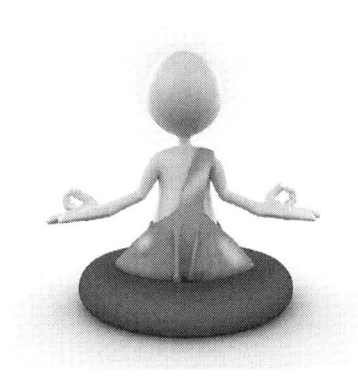

I practiced Bikram Yoga. Each class contains the same set of 26 yoga poses. Each pose is done twice, and then there is a rest. The instructor guides you with their voice throughout the class. Just listen and follow the directions.

When I first started the 90-minute hot yoga class, I would go home and sleep like a rock for 3-4 hours. It took me several months to figure out why I was so exhausted. Focusing on the instructor's words for 90 minutes was like climbing Mount Kilimanjaro.

Strength

A study at Tuft University demonstrated that, after only 8 weeks of weight training, elderly clients showed a vast

Concussion Recovery

improvement in balance, muscle tone, energy level and bone density.[viii]

Express Brain Builders *Will try*

Although many different exercises have been developed for the brain and its balance, I have chosen only a few for this book. I have included the rest in my video so that you can follow along.

These Express Brain Builders are designed to make a healthier brain. The following exercises are quick to do and form part of a longer series explained in the Personal Workbook section.

Before you start, drink a glass of water. Keep yourself hydrated.

1. Put your thumb under your ear lobe and spread your fingers above the ear. Keeping your thumb stiff, tap your fingers on the area around the top of the ear for about 30 seconds.
2. With your arms crossed and feet shoulder length apart, move your hands up to your ears and massage your whole ear. While massaging your ears, simply do squats to the best of your ability for 5- 10 minutes. Try this three times a day, perhaps before each meal, as a reminder.
3. Grasp your hands together with your thumbs up.
4. Hold your arms straight out in front of you, and then draw an infinity sign, (i.e., a sideways figure eight) in the air in front of you.
5. With your eyes fixed on your thumbs, follow their movement with your eyes, keeping your head straight.

Concussion Recovery

6. Follow the movement of your thumbs for 2-3 minutes, in each direction. This helps to balance the right and left hemispheres of your brain. If you are too sore to do this for yourself, simply ask a friend to draw the shape in the air with a pencil, and then follow the shape with your eyes.

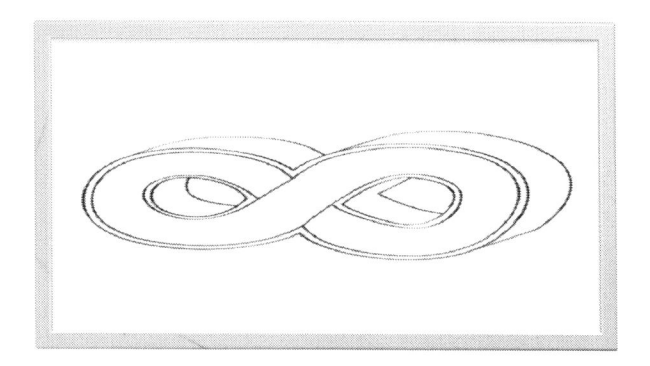

7. Finally, we come to De-Switching the brain by Dr. Doepp.[ix] This has 3 parts and takes a total of 1 minute to do. It is best practiced 3 times a day, perhaps again just before or after mealtime.

a. Cross your arms, placing your thumb on the top inside corner of your brow bone near to where your eyebrows meet. With your thumb firmly planted, use your fingers to massage your eyebrow area along your eyeball socket bone for 20 seconds.

b. With your arms crossed again, massage your ears with your thumb on the outside of your ear lobe and your fingers on the inside. Gently massage the whole ear for 20 seconds.

c. Place one baby finger on the bridge between your lip and nose. Place the other baby finger just below the bone beneath your lips. Rock back and forth, gently massaging the bone for 10 seconds, and then switch fingers and massage for another 10 seconds. This will help with your connections in the brain, giving you heightened alertness throughout the day.

Exercise:

What do you do when you hurt all over and you cannot focus?

- Try an Epsom salts bath.
- Breathe deeply and practice flexing your muscles so that the fluids flow to the brain.
- Visualize white light and try to run it along your spine, up one side and down the other.
- Go for a walk in the fresh air. Flushing the system with clean air is like steam cleaning a carpet!

In Summary

There are many techniques that can help to get your brain back on track. Some may work well for you. Others may not work for you, even after a 6-week trial.

Keep your exercises fun, well rounded and regular! Even if we huff and puff and have to take many breaks, fresh oxygenated blood is flowing to all parts of our brain.

I look forward to sharing this with you in the video so that you can follow along at home. No matter how you are or where you are, I encourage you to start today.

Mental Exercise

Right now, mental exercise is as important for you as physical exercise.

Simply put, the brain has two hemispheres. The right hemisphere, which is creative, controls the left side of the body. The left hemisphere controls the right side of the body and is in charge of math and problem solving.

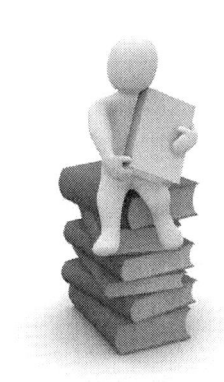

After the accident, I had trouble with my memory. I could not remember numbers. So I needed to start with baby steps to develop those pathways again.

Although I tried many different games and techniques, Electronic Sudoku was my favorite game for developing memory recall. I played as much as 4 hours a day. The effort of concentration was so great that I would have to nap afterward. I took tiny steps of progress.

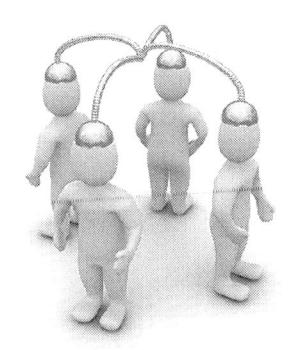

It took me nearly 2 years of playing Sudoku on the computer before I learned to do it right. Then it took me another year before I felt capable of working in paperback form! I still prefer the electronic Sudoku because the game allows you to take up to 5 guesses before you lose the game and have to start it again. Plus, there is no track record of mistakes!

I found that my ability to figure things out was closely related to my level of fatigue or stress. There were days when I wasn't able to figure the game out at all, and then, the next day, after a good sleep, I was dynamite at playing it. This was a benefit that I hadn't expected. I became more aware of myself and recognized how my performance would vary. I didn't have to be at the top of my game all of the time.

I tried other games as well, such as Nintendo, Big Brain, Brain Age and Brain Age2. But I prefer Brain Age2 because the graphics were better and I was able to chart my progress.

There are other games and sites on the Internet, such as Luminosity.com, which is a very good site that is similar to the Nintendo games. Although the games were trying at times, I did notice a difference in my ability.

You will need a considerable amount of determination in order to succeed at these activities. But you must persevere.

Keep your mind active with thinking games, such as these:

- Crossword
- Word search
- Scrabble

Concussion Recovery

If you have never tried these activities, learn to knit, fish, play an instrument or learn a new language. A craft or art project will stimulate new ideas and foster new neural pathways.

Personally, I built a rock fountain in my yard. I filled the pond with gold fish, and then spent the rest of the summer trying to keep the raccoons from eating my fish! It was a fun project that stretched my abilities, even if they were reduced at the time.

Many people ask about the role of television in the recovery of a brain-injured person. Television often offers too much stimulation. It is a passive activity. But the stimulating effect of television can be overwhelming. Limit the time you spend watching television and choose programs for their uplifting content.

With a bruised brain, we are still sculpting a new piece of art. The clay is still wet. We are a work in progress.

Above all things, be kind to yourself.

Massage

Massage is so enjoyable and it offers gentle alignment of the physical and neurological systems. There are many styles and forms of massage. So feel

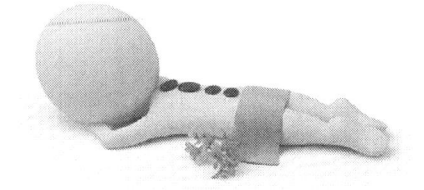

Concussion Recovery

free to explore what type works best for you.

Reflexology is a system of hand, foot and ear massage, which you can practice on yourself. A professional will most likely do a better job. However, you can do little harm to yourself. To stimulate the brain meridians, massage the big toes, thumb tips and lobes of the ears. There are even reflexology maps of emotions that you may want to research on your own to help you along your journey.

Acupuncture and therapeutic massage by a registered massage therapist can open up blocked passageways, de-stress the body and leave you with a greater sense of well being.

To bolster the effect of massage, encourage your practitioner to use magnesium oil, instead of regular oil. Magnesium oil melts sore muscles, stimulates the neurological and muscular systems and helps with dehydration. There are many wonderful side effects of magnesium and using the oil is just one more way of ensuring that you are giving your brain everything possible for it to grow and heal.

I encourage you to use massage as another tool to stimulate the brain.

Concussion Recovery

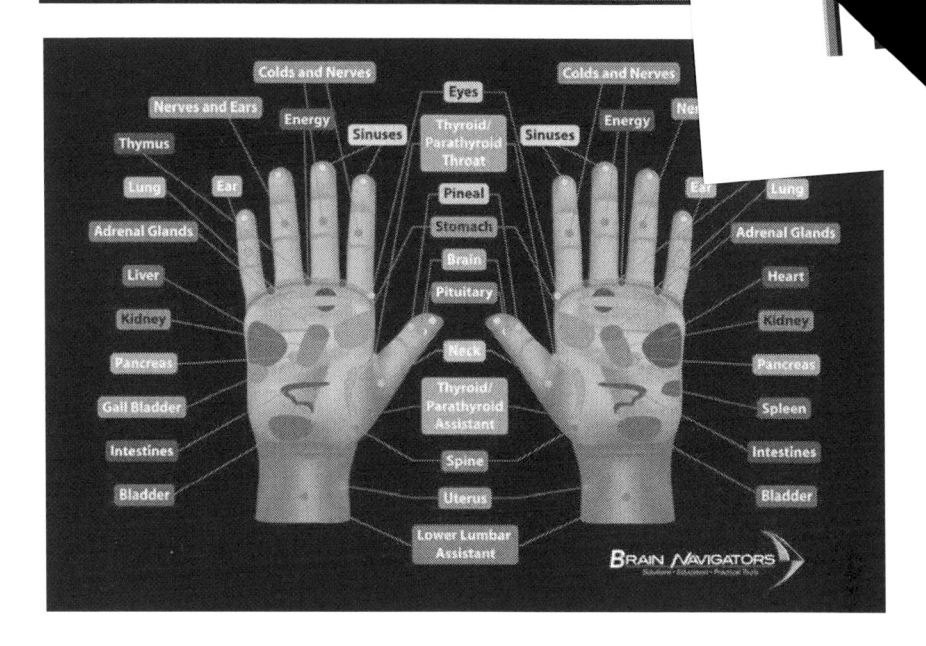

These are the areas of the ear. Each ear is different. A massage will greatly boost your energy level - physically, mentally and emotionally. Focus on massaging the lobe.

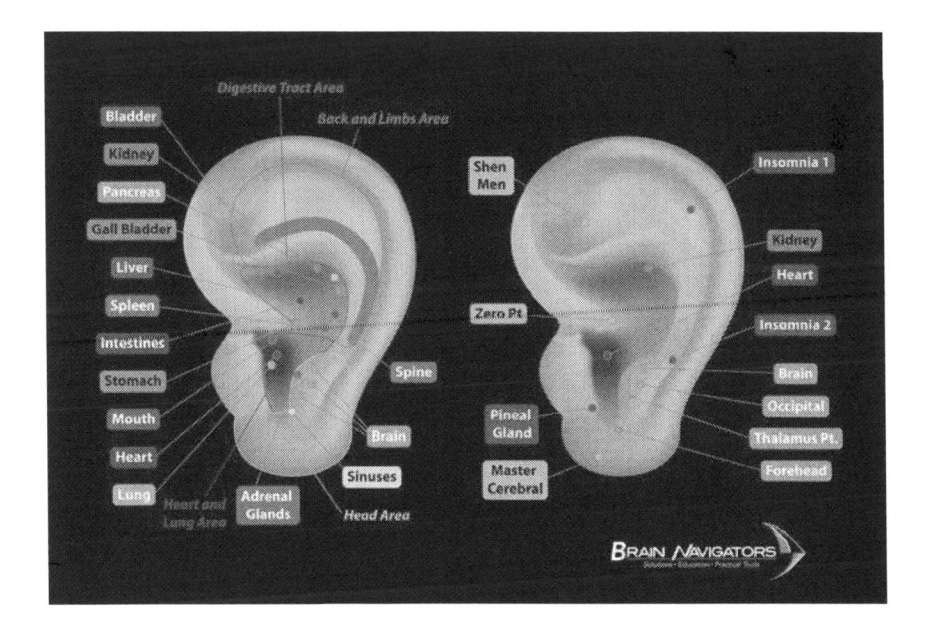

Concussion Recovery

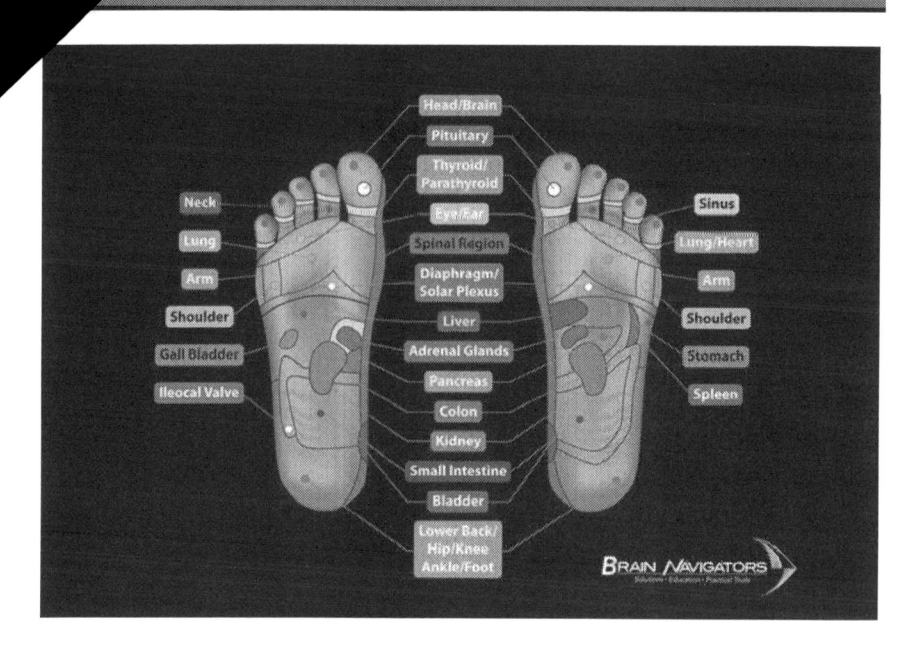

Boundaries

Boundaries are our personal rules. They are our own personal `Ten Commandments.' Boundaries are our fortress.

Even when we are healthy, boundaries are difficult to set. With an injury to the brain, our boundaries become blurred. We become gullible, vulnerable and easily persuaded.

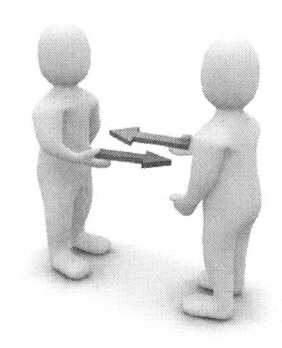

Because our injury cannot be seen, we are often in denial about the degree of severity of the injury. As an example, a doctor who had suffered a head injury continued to practice, despite his injury. One day, his colleagues pulled him aside, examined him and sent him home.

If a doctor who has all of the training in the world can experience a head injury, without knowing it, then you shouldn't feel bad or beat yourself up if you are one of the many people who have fallen through the cracks.

Our abilities to set boundaries and to understand social rules fluctuate. When we are well rested and feeling little stress, we can cope. But, if you add stress or sleeplessness to that same scenario, we cannot function. This is why a brain injury is so confusing.

Still, we need to recreate and reconnect our boundaries. There is no clear rule to follow about re-establishing your boundaries. Everyone is different.

There is a wonderful book called, *Feelings Buried Alive Never Die,* by Karol K. Truman. This book helps by redirecting our brain and ourselves toward the type of person we would be proud to be. Over a period of several weeks, we simply tell our brains what it is that we want to become. (However, keep in mind that, under healthy conditions, it takes six weeks to form a new habit.)

One of the methods explained in the book must be prepared in advance. Write a 'cheat sheet' with 2-24 words of what you would like to change. Some examples could be:

- I choose to make wise choices. I feel like I make wise choices. I am making wise choices.
- I am happy. I feel happy. I am.

Now, take a long walk in nature.

Centre yourself and take 6 good breathes. Breathe in through your nose and blow out through your mouth, as hard as you can.

As you walk, continuously repeat the words on the 'cheat sheet' that you have prepared. It is best to say those words aloud because they resonate throughout your body.

As the conductor of your orchestra, you create the world in which you want to live. Your words will change as these words become your world.

It is okay to go back to these core words, from time to time. You are creating. You are directing. You are building a new brain.

Give it time. Trust yourself. You are uploading the new version of Windows - your windows.

Letting Go

When we learn to stop trying to duplicate our past life and start to create a new life, we really begin to grow.

Let go!

Stop the struggle!

We need to mourn the past, and then move on.

Embrace the moment. If we accept things for what they are, we can rejoice in the present. We need to wallow in compassion and empathy for ourselves.

Finances

How are your finances? *Manageable*

This is often the first question that I ask my clients. Invariably they answer, *"Fine. Why do you ask?"* Later in the discussion, the lights come on and the client realizes that they paid a bill three times and are in overdraft.

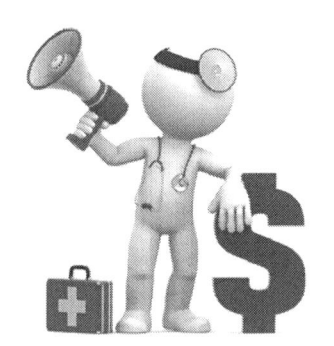

With a head injury, you are more vulnerable and gullible. So delay making any major decisions. If something is a great deal today, it will be a great deal tomorrow, and there always will be another great deal.

Hold off making any type of financial decision. The ability to reason and set boundaries is not as sound as it was in the past. Buy only the essentials.

Put everything on hold. If you can, find someone whom you can trust emphatically and assign them the responsibility of attending to your financial matters.

Broken boundaries and addictions go hand in hand. So you may become highly addicted to buying jewelry or cars. Be careful.

I once had a client who spent all of her money on a bracelet, and then borrowed money to buy trinkets for the bracelet. She had never bought herself anything nice and, now with a brain injury, she splurged. She had no money left with which to pay her mortgage or buy food. She had no boundaries when it came to money.

We might be denying the fact that our brain is still sick or damaged. We may try to hide our mistakes. We might even forget our mistakes. Little errors add up!

At this point in your life, you need to put 100 percent of your focus on growing your brain.

Structure

Just when I thought everything was well and it was time to get back to leading a productive life, my brain was acting up and throwing temper tantrums! I didn't want to work. I wanted to procrastinate. I felt no urgency. My brain had been introduced to a new sense of time. It had learned to relax and luxuriate in life.

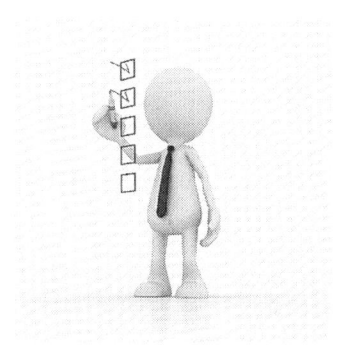

My next step in my recovery was to learn balance!

I have had to learn to balance my time, consciously structuring it to include healthy amounts of time for sleep, play, work, creativity, rejuvenation, meditation and friendship.

Concussion Recovery

As difficult as it is to make and follow a schedule, I believe we need to be much more cognizant of structure and timetables. We need to buy a calendar or a Day-Timer, and we need to use it. Find a way to build a consistent schedule so that Wednesday can be 'Friends Day' and, on Monday, Wednesday and Friday, there is time slotted in for exercise. We need concrete tangible reminders because hours can slip into days, and then days can slip into months.

[Handwritten note: Outlook - use all the time. Blackberry!]

Music

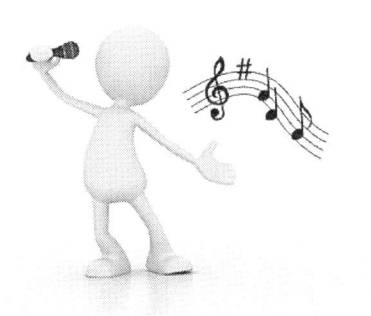

— exceedingly — works over(?)

The beauty about the music and the brain is that music is processed by the entire brain.

Think of this...

At Boston's Beth Israel Deaconess Medical Centre, researchers have found that the brain actually grows during musical training, in the same way that other muscles in the body respond to exercise![x]

Music can activate the attention network on both sides of the brain, whereas spoken word activities only activate areas in the left hemisphere.

Music is exactly what the injured brain needs. Why?

- The structure of the music helps to re-organize the structure of the brain. Classical music, like Bach, Beethoven and Mozart, is most effective.
- The rhythm of the music helps improve motor skills. When you tap, walk, dance and keep time to the music, you are able to respond to life better. Studies show that Alzheimer's patients, who interacted with music, were happier and had better memories.

Obviously, the lyrics also need to be carefully scrutinized. Anything containing abusive or derogatory comments should not come anywhere around an injured brain because you are inputting thoughts, even though you may not be conscious of all of them. Positive, kind, upbeat music that brings joy or a smile to your heart is best.

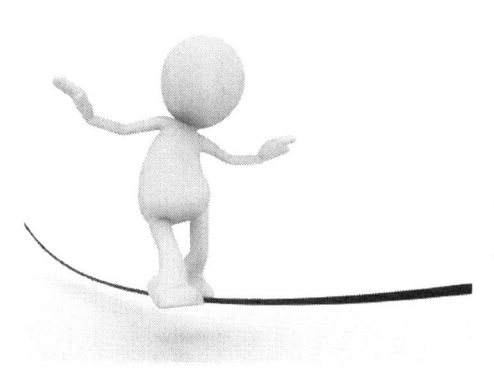

Listen to music that relaxes you. This is another tool for your toolbox. Guess what? With music, you just need to sit back and relax... no thinking, no doing, just ENJOY!

Spiritual Aspects

The work of scientists, Dr. Jill Bolte Taylor and Carolon Leaf PhD., is amazing. Their research connects the brain to the evolution of spirituality, and our reconnection with the universe and source. We are multi-dimensional beings.

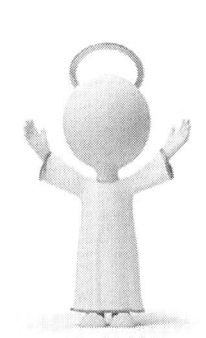

The knock on our noggins definitely reroutes our thinking and creates a newly evolving person that is more in tune with the world around us. Our brain injury has given us an opportunity to transform into more perceptive caring people. We can balance out our right and left hemispheres, balancing task management with caring.

It took me having an accident before I was able to be successful at prayer. As I close my eyes, I remember to be thankful for all of the wonderful things in my life. There are very few nights when I do not say the Lord's Prayer and ask for guidance. I'm not a really religious person, so this is a big step for me.

When there are things in my life that I do not like, I may mention them. However, I assume that these areas of discomfort have been accomplished.

For example, if your memory is weak, you might say, "*Thank you for showing me how to remember names again.*" For walking, you might say, *"Thank you for my increased coordination."*

Whether it is in yoga, meditation, church, walking in nature or fly-fishing, taking the time to turn your troubles over to someone else is a wonderful relief. It helps to clean out the clutter from the brain.

Prayer quiets the brain chatter. It is important for starting the process of thinking positively and making your desires known to the Universe. Prayer is a time for solitude, to let go of the old and to invite your new world into yourself.

Prior to my accident, there was nothing in my life that said God, Jesus, Spirit, Jehovah or Buddha. But, now, I know that there is something more. What you call it does not matter. But talking to it does.

In my healing, I discovered a phrase that gave me an intense sense of well being and peace. This phrase helped me to release a lot of negativity that had been building up and, somewhere along the way, it replaced the can't do's with the can do's. I do not know if it will work for you:

Jesus wept. All is well. God is God. Thy will be done. I am. You are.

When you are lying in pain, there is not much to do, except pray for what you would like to create or for where you would like to be. Explore. Soul searching is part of brain rebuilding.

Sex and Intimacy

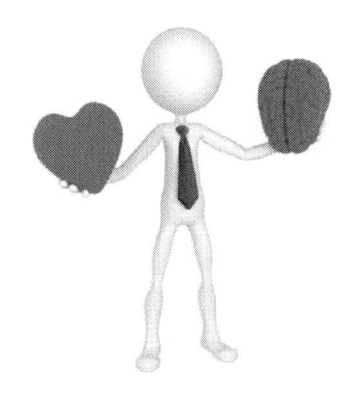

Of all the topics in the world, our conversations rarely include sex and intimacy. But they are a reality of life. It is why you and I are here. Intimacy is an expression of caring, loving and sharing that we show each other. It helps us to feel wanted and needed.

We need intimacy. But the journey of the brain injured is often a very personal, solo journey. The concept of sharing is difficult because even everyday tasks are exhausting. The need for intimacy may drop very low on the priority list.

The lack of desire or the unrestrained interest of the brain-injured person, as well as the level of anxiety around the subject, are determined by the degree and type of brain injury. I know that, when my head would go into overdrive from too much stimulation or if mind chatter was rampant, my desire for intimacy was as great as wanting to wear a bikini at the Arctic Circle in January.

Sex can be aligned very closely with music because it engages nearly the entire brain. The art of intimacy or the act of lovemaking is definitely a multi-tasking skill that requires the organizational ability of the left side of the brain and the feeling ability of the right side. Damage to either, or both sides, will affect your ability and desire for intimacy and sex.

On the other hand, the need for sex can be addictive and promiscuity is a possibility because our boundaries are broken, and our personal values of right and wrong are being re-arranged. While the brain is in recovery, we are vulnerable. We may not be able to recognize danger because our ability to discern has been damaged. Caution is needed.

As the brain heals and balances it self, desires and abilities will change. Sex and intimacy may not be the same. If we understand our bodies and listen to our intuition, we make our lives more fulfilling.

The Healing Team

The brain is still such a wonder that even sophisticated machines are not as sensitive as human beings and human techniques.

There are many types of healing that are available to us when we are rebuilding our brains. Each technique will have something to offer, whether or not you decide to continue with that particular type of healing.

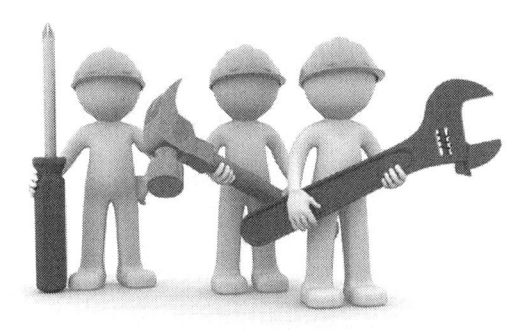

Let's get practical! Have you tried the following?

- Acupuncture ✓
- Acupressure
- Aromatherapy
- Brainwave Biofeedback
- Chinese Herbalist
- Chiropractor ✓
- Clinical psycho neurophysiology
- Cranial sacral therapy

Concussion Recovery

- Geo-tran
- Healing touch
- Herbs
- Jin-shin Do
- Massage therapy ✓
- Nutritional Counseling
- Naturopath
- Neurophysiologist
- Neurotherapeutic techniques
- Osteopath
- Personal trainer ✓
- Psychologist ✓
- Scar Tissue Relief
- Tap touching
- Visualization

I encourage you to find the healing arts and the practitioners that are perfect for you.

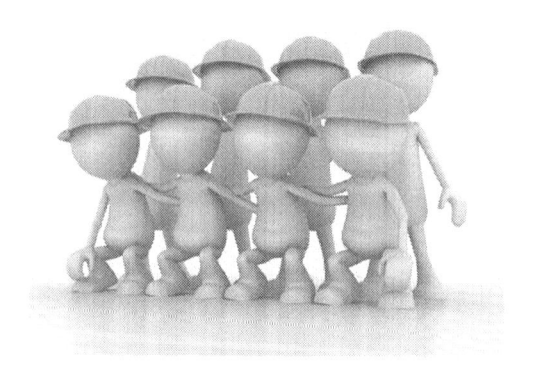

In Closing

Looking back, the accident probably saved my life. It gave me the time to look at myself, to face my weaknesses and to overcome them. It has given me the chance to be grateful for the things that I might have just passed right by.

This may sound frivolous but in hindsight I wish I had not fretted and stressed in fear of not recovering. I wish I had enjoyed the journey more.

Yes, it was a terrible journey sometimes, one that no one else should go through alone, but I feel that I am wiser and more empathetic. I appreciate nature. I take time to really listen.

Without a shadow of a doubt, our brains are INCREDIBLE and the plasticity is AMAZING! When you release the image of what your life was and your new life is embraced, recovery begins and joy sprouts out of the most unexpected things. I believe that nothing is taken without something greater given.

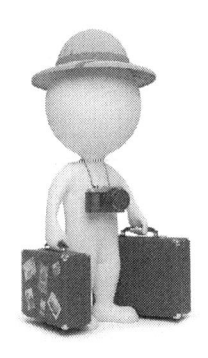

You are not alone. Trust your intuition, even if it speaks in a soft voice.

Let me know where your journey takes you.

Concussion Recovery

Appendix A: Creation of Personal Work Book

Now is time for your reflections, plans and even some soul searching. You are your own best advocate and healer. I encourage you to be as thorough as possible.

Turn to the last page of this workbook and draw a picture of your life now. Draw how you feel. Include any symbols that are significant for you. Call this one, "Where I have been."

Next, on the previous page, draw a picture of how you would like to feel. I want you to see your dreams. Put in as much detail as possible and date your drawing. You don't have to be a maestro of art. Be free. Call this one, "Where I am going."

Concussion Recovery

I_____, do solemnly swear that I am the conductor of my brain. It is my responsibility as conductor of my brain to stimulate all parts of my brain no matter how disobedient they may be. I _____ am the conductor of my Brain, its thoughts and actions therefore I will train my Brain to be a winner and play the music melody of peace, prosperity, harmony and tranquility throughout my life.

What I am most proud of myself for.....

1. _____
2. _____
3. _____

What would I like to change about me right now?

1. _____
2. _____
3. _____

What can I do to become the person I want to be?

1. _____
2. _____
3. _____

Concussion Recovery

Mind Chatter

Every time your mind starts to chatter, say, "I release double minded. I compute. I am single minded. I am integrated minded. I am whole minded."

When my mind chatters to itself, the best ways for me to stop it is:
1. Go for run
2. Drive/work on car
3. Drink beer.

What are MY triggers for depression?
1. Caden's Care
2. inability to function pre-injury
3. _____

When I start to feel depressed I feel like:
1. Quiet
2. to be alone
3. Don't care about much

Concussion Recovery

MY action plan to fight depression is:

1. _____
2. _____
3. _____

What makes me happy and peaceful?

1. Janine
2. Kids
3. Care driving, working

How can I bring more of what makes me happy and peaceful into my life?

1. _____
2. _____
3. _____

Concussion Recovery

Brain Builders

1. Put your thumb under your ear lobe and spread your fingers above the ear. Keeping your thumb stiff, tap your fingers on the area around the top of the ear for about 30 seconds.

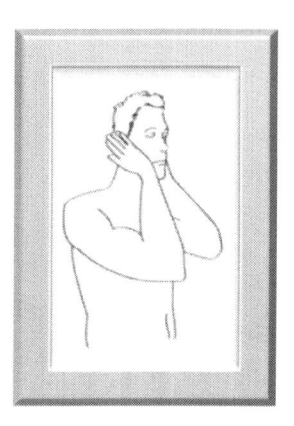

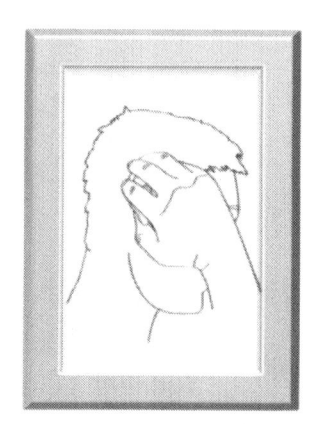

2. With your arms crossed and feet shoulder length apart, move your hands up to your ears and massage your whole ear. While massaging your ears, simply do squats to the best of your ability for 5- 10 minutes. Try this three times a day, perhaps before each meal, as a reminder.

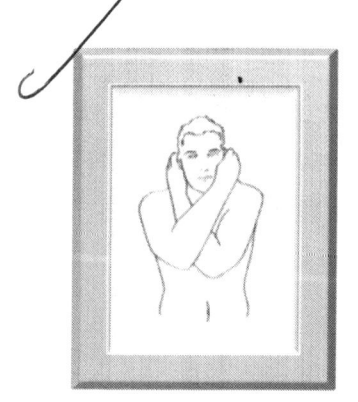

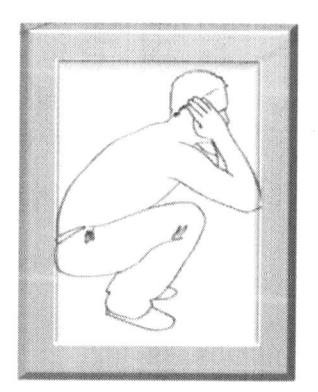

Concussion Recovery

3. Grasp your hands together with your thumbs up.

   a. Hold your arms straight out in front of you, and then draw an infinity sign, (i.e., a sideways figure eight) in the air in front of you.
   b. With your eyes fixed on your thumbs, follow their movement with your eyes, keeping your head straight.
   c. Follow the movement of your thumbs for 2-3 minutes, in each direction. This helps to balance the right and left hemispheres of your brain. If you are too sore to do this for yourself, simply ask a friend to draw the shape in the air with a pencil, and then follow the shape with your eyes.

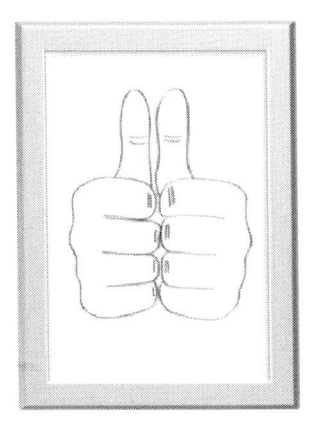

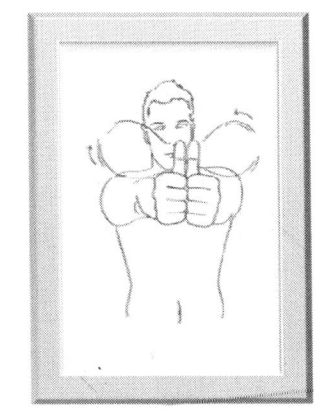

   3a   3b

Concussion Recovery

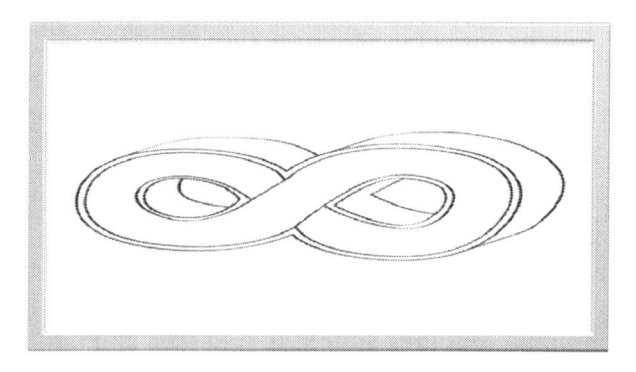

3c

4. De-Switching the brain by Dr. Doepp. This has 3 parts and takes a total of 1 minute to do. It is best practiced 3 times a day, perhaps again just before or after mealtime.

    a. Cross your arms, placing your thumb on the top inside corner of your brow bone near to where your eyebrows meet. With your thumb firmly planted, use your fingers to massage your eyebrow area along your eyeball socket bone for 20 seconds.

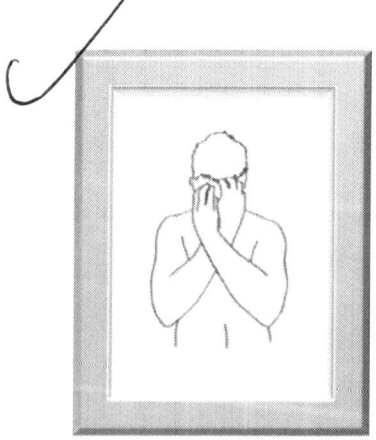

Massage eye brow area

Concussion Recovery

b. With your arms crossed again, massage your ears with your thumb on the outside of your ear lobe and your fingers on the inside. Gently massage the whole ear for 20 seconds.

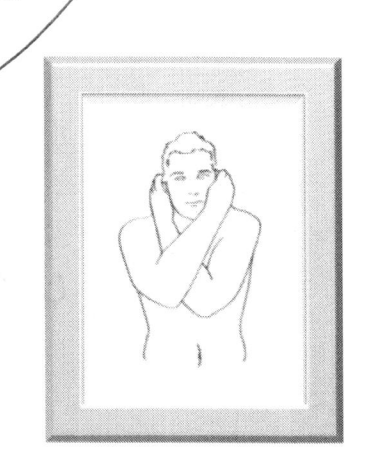

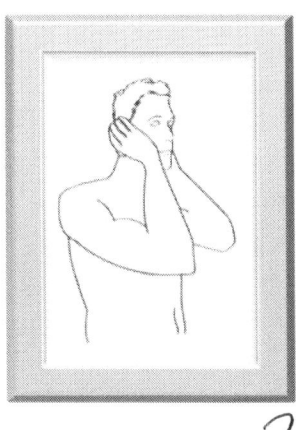

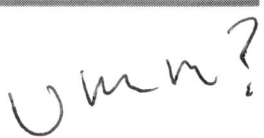

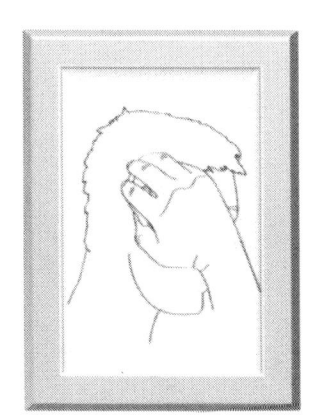

Umm?

Concussion Recovery

Massage Ears

    c. Place one baby finger on the bridge between your lip and nose. Place the other baby finger just below the bone beneath your lips. Rock back and forth, gently massaging the bone for 10 seconds, and then switch fingers and massage for another 10 seconds. This will help with your connections in the brain, giving you heightened alertness throughout the day.

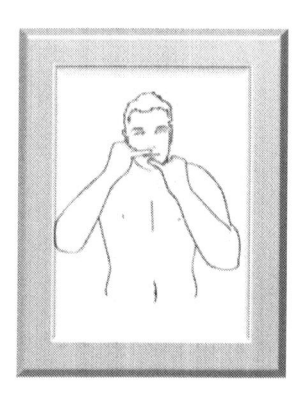

Good, now you need just 5 minutes to complete the rest of the set.

Concussion Recovery

5. Touch and hear- Awakens hearing.

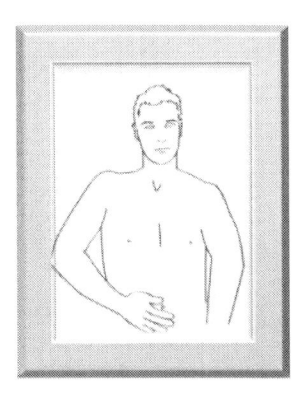

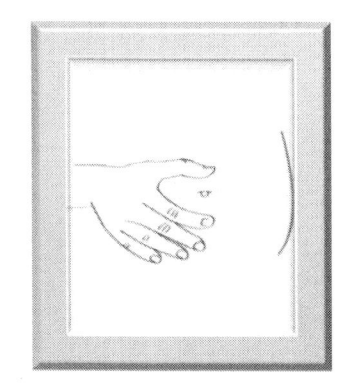

   Put your left finger in your navel, and place your right hand 2 inches from the navel and 1 ½' down from the navel so your thumb and forefinger draw a C around your navel. Hold to the count of 20.

6. Touch crown of head- Draws attention to present time and stops the mind from wandering.

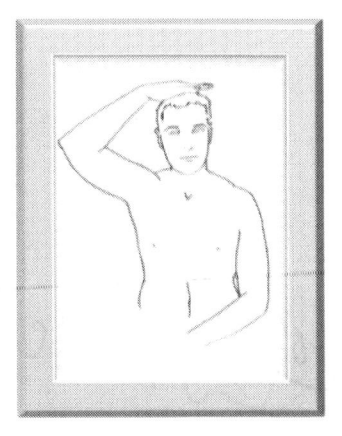

Concussion Recovery

Cover the soft spot on the crown of your head with the palm of your right hand for the count of 20.

Repeat the same action with your left palm. Hold for the count of 20.

7. Cross and touch back of head- Activates brain and clears fear.

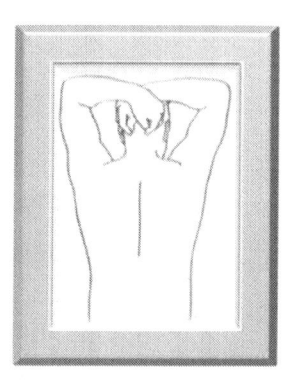

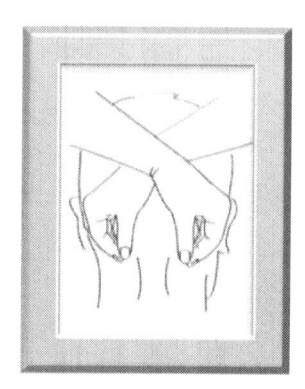

Make a cone with fingers of right hand and touch left bone at base of skull. Simultaneously, cone fingers of left hand and touch the corresponding right bone at base of skull. Hold for 20 seconds.

Reverse action. (This means that the first time, the right arm will be on top and the second time, the left arm will be on top.) Hold for 20 seconds.

Concussion Recovery

8. Switch on-Restores balance and clears electrical system.

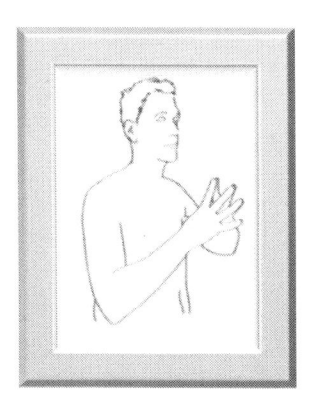

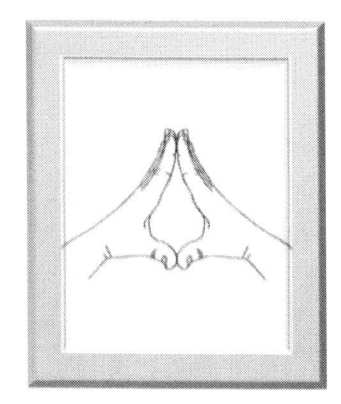

   At the same time, touch tips of all fingers and both thumbs together in front of you. Hold for the count of 20.

9. Cross and touch shoulders- Balances positive and negative charges and polarity.

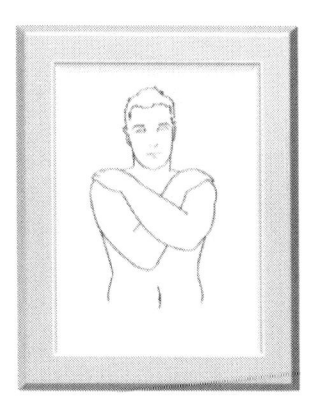

   Place the right hand on left shoulder and left hand on right shoulder. Hold 20 seconds. Reverse action. Hold 20 seconds.

Concussion Recovery

10. Cross and touch back of neck- Restores centeredness and clears anger. This is like giving your self a hug.

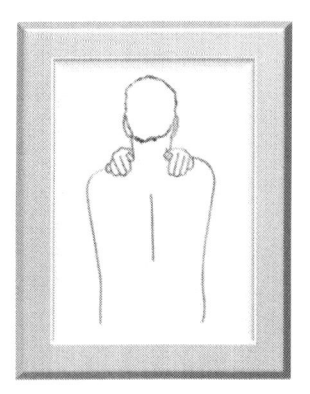

Place right hand on left back of neck where it connects to the shoulder and left hand on right back of neck where it attaches to the shoulder. Hold for 20 seconds. Reverse so the other arm is on the top and hold for 20 seconds.

Concussion Recovery

THE EXERCISES BELOW ARE WITH ALL FOUR FINGERS RESTING ON THE THUMB PAD OF EACH HAND. THIS IS CALLED CONED HANDS.

11. Cross and touch at hairline- Helps with mind chatter and restores color hues. Use when you feeling angry.

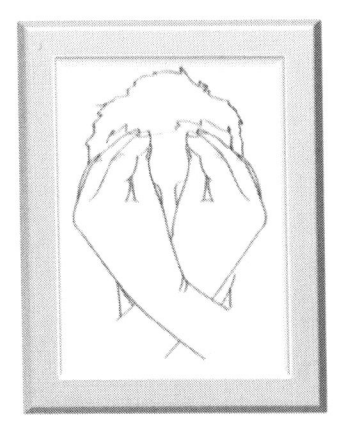

Cone your fingers. Touch the right hand on the left side of the forehead at hairline. Touch the left hand on the right side of the hairline and count to 20. Reverse the action so the other arm is on top. Hold for 20 again.

12. Cross and touch at mid forehead just above the center of your eyes- This will help to clear mind chatter.

Concussion Recovery

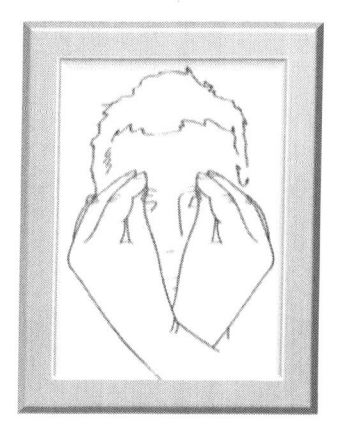

With your coned fingers, place the right cone above the left eyeball mid forehead and the left coned fingers above the right eye mid forehead. Hold for 20. Reverse the action. That means you slide the right hand out and place it over the left arm at the same spots as before, for 20.

13. Cross and touch at the naval- This will clear rage, terror and hate.

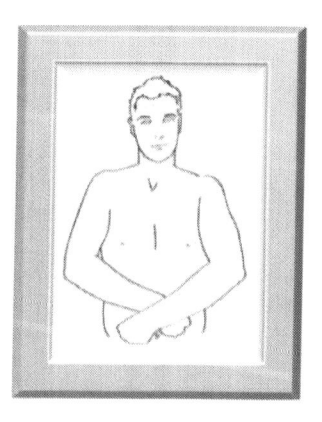

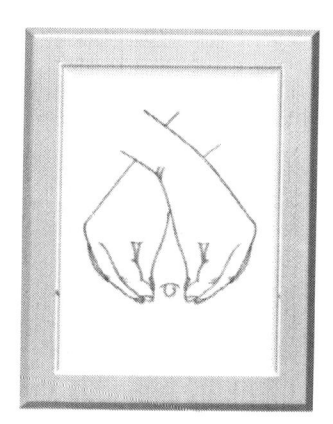

Concussion Recovery

With coned fingers, have the right hand touch the left side of naval and the left hand touch the right side of the naval for a count of 20. Reverse the arms so the left arm is closest to the body. Hold for a count of 20.

14. Cross and touch at the crown of the head- This helps to clear trauma from your body.

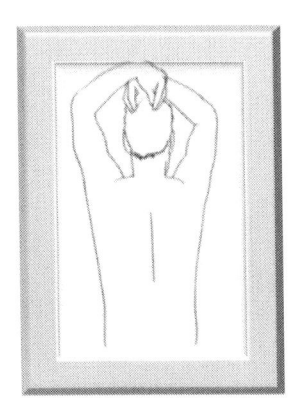

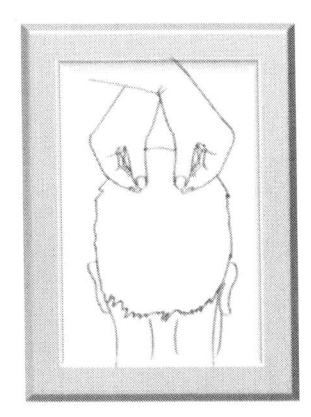

With coned fingers, the right hand goes on the crown of the head (1 ½ "from soft spot) and the left goes to the right side of the soft spot. Hold to the count of 20. Reverse by crossing your left hand over your right. Hold for 20.

Concussion Recovery

15. Cross and touch at Thymus gland- This will help to clear shock, anxiety, destruction of self.

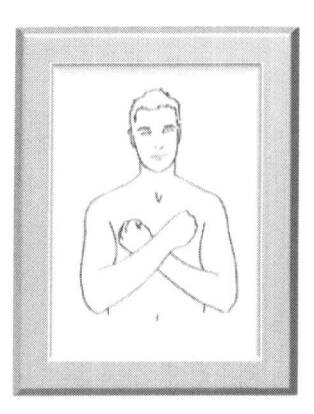

Cone fingers of right hand and touch left side of the thymus gland, 2' down from the top sternum (just below the prominent bone in the sternum). At the same time, place coned left hand on the right side of the thymus gland and hold for a count of 20. Reverse by lifting the right arm so it is on top of the left arm Hold for 20.

Concussion Recovery

16. In-Vision- Create the world you desire!

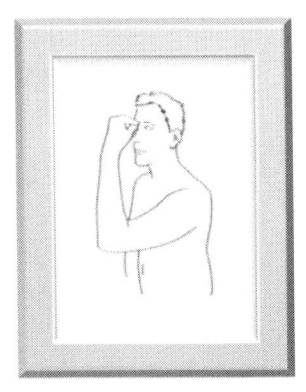

Cone the fingers of your dominant hand and place them on the pineal gland between the eyes. Hold until you are finished visualizing all of your dreams and desires.

The best times to remember Brain Builders are:

1. _____

2. _____

3. _____

Music integrates both sides of the brain. I can introduce music into my life by:

1. _____

2. _____

3. _____

Concussion Recovery

I can challenge the creative side of my brain by:

1. _____

2. _____

3. _____

	9	3	1		5	6	4	
7								5
5		1	2		9	3		7
2								3
	3	6	9		7	5	2	
9								1
3		2	4		8	1		9
6								4
	4	7	3		2	8	5	

1		5			2		3	
	3	8	7	5	6	4	1	
	2		9		8		3	
		9			1			
	4		6		2		7	
	1	3	4	9	5	7	8	
7		4			3			6

Concussion Recovery

```
P Z X W X S N G N S Q W X Z
K L X Q U U C O K D T G G S
T W A O Y P D D V R L A K U
O D W N N L S Q N A R F R N
I F M X E U S U S D P T H A
U A I W W T J F W N X D K R
G Z L I I O S Q E S S X G U
J R M A P L Z P I S D C M Q
X E S A J B T G U Q O L T F
Y T N V R U E N R U T A S E
L I M G N S E P U U E G E T
S P R E S V Z K Q W W K X A
L U H T R A E G G F W G E A
V J A M E R C U R Y Z Z H C
```

VENUS	SATURN
URANUS	MARS
NEPTUNE	MERCURY
EARTH	STAR
JUPITER	PLANETS
PLUTO	NOVA

I can best challenge my analytical brain by:

1. _____

2. _____

3. _____

Exercise is good because it gets the blood flowing to the brain and encourages growth. The best exercise for me is:

1. _____

2. _____

3. _____

Concussion Recovery

What are my barriers to exercising?

1. _____

2. _____

3. _____

How can I best overcome my barriers? What works best for me?

1. _____

2. _____

3. _____

How can I add exercise to my schedule?

1. _____

2. _____

3. _____

Concussion Recovery

I am able to commit to myself exercise daily by:

	Mon	Tues	Wed	Thu	Fri	Sat	Sun
Aerobic Type Time							
Strength Type Time							
Poise Type Time							
Flexibility Type Time							

Not Therapeutic

Bikram (Hot Yoga) heals the body and retrains the brain. Heat soothes and detoxes so that I can move easily and be more flexible. I learn to pay attention for longer time spans and my body becomes aligned so fluids flow with ease to the brain. I become smarter. My brain gets a good work out and my body heals. If there is no Bikram Yoga available to me, I can align my body myself by:

Concussion Recovery

1. _____

   (Lie down on stomach head to one side, toes pointed in and breathe for 1 min then change other direction. You might need a heating pad or hot water bottle for this.)

2. _____

3. _____

While exercising, I use these Brain Builders to become the conductor of my brain: (Remember, if you are feeling negative, use the opposite words to re-route your brain: I am the boss. I am happy. My mind works perfectly. Etc.)

1. _____

2. _____

3. _____

To slow my mind and help to repair my body and brain, I visualize:

1. _____

2. _____

3. _____

Concussion Recovery

Rebuilding the Brain Chart

Plan your week ahead. Commit at least some time every day to each of these categories, increasing time as you feel is right.

	Mon	Tues	Wed	Tu	Fri	Sat	Sun
Physical exercise							
Mental exercise							
Emotional laughing							
Brain Builder exercises							

Laughing is good for me because it brings more oxygen into the brain, stimulating all areas. It helps to keep me positive and happy. I can invite more laughter into my life by:

1. _Drinking beer_
2. _Smoking pot_
3. _Not caring about how F'd up I am._

Einstein said, "Why should I remember anything that I can look up?" He didn't remember anything that he could look up and

Concussion Recovery

kept his mind free for new ideas. If he wanted to remember something he would simply write it down. If I need to remember something, what is the best way for me to remember?

1. _____
2. _____
3. _____

Nutrition:

When we have a broken leg, we do not run a marathon, as we do not play basketball with broken arms. We must nourish our brain back to health. The food we once ate prior to the incident may not be being digested as effectively as before... it is baby steps! This is a new world we are creating and opportunities are abundant.

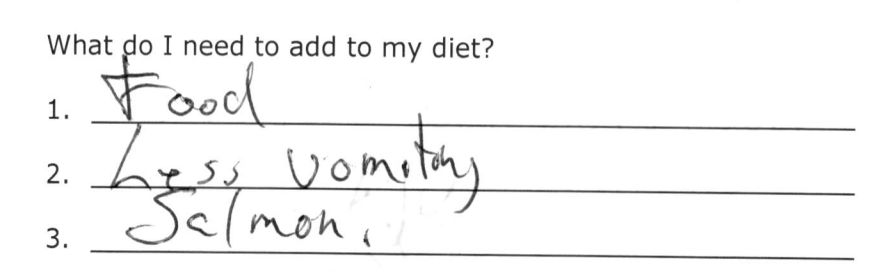

What do I need to add to my diet?
1. Food
2. Less vomiting
3. Salmon,

Concussion Recovery

What do I need to subtract from my diet?
1. Ain't
2. Garlic — Ofactory — pain
3. _____

What was the most surprising thing I learned about diet?
1. Nothing surprising —
2. a lot of prep for little eat.
3. _____

Structure: Because our brain has been shaken and the concept of time is nearly non-existent for some of us, there is a need to bring back some structure. As with every injury, there are different areas we need to work on. Once we know our strengths and weaknesses, we can keep ourselves in check until we are more balanced.

What can we do to put structure into our lives?
1. Become a Nazi supremacist
2. Jet berg me again — Please!
3. Not be a dependant invalid

Concussion Recovery

How do we keep ourselves in check?
1. Thank Jesus - ah ha ha ha!
2. Know - I can fix this
3. Sleep

Do we need a buddy to help us?
1. No - I have 10 "buddies"
2. shows up to baby sit me.
3. go away - stress - embarrassing

My strengths are:
1. Throwing the couch.
2. Lifting Janine - one arm
3. Telling her. I am in here.

My areas of concern are:
1. Will I be me
2. Janine - so worried.
3. Feel responsible for Fall.

Concussion Recovery

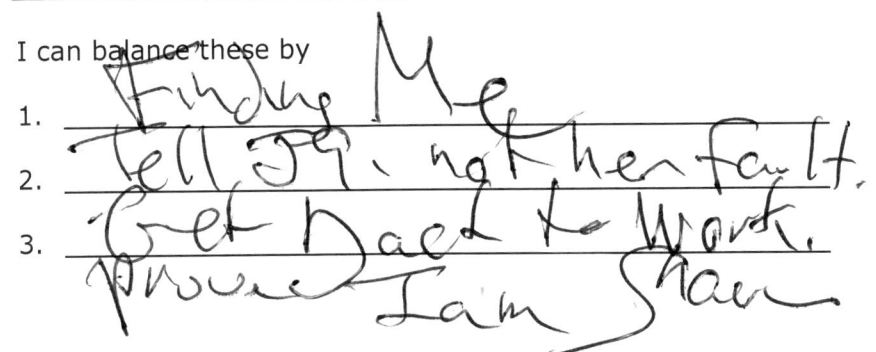

I can balance these by

1. _Finding Me_
2. _Telling not her fault._
3. _Get back to work._
   Prove I am Shawn

In the final stages of recovery, we need structure to keep us on track. This exercise is not recommended nor will work until you feel you are ready for the next step!

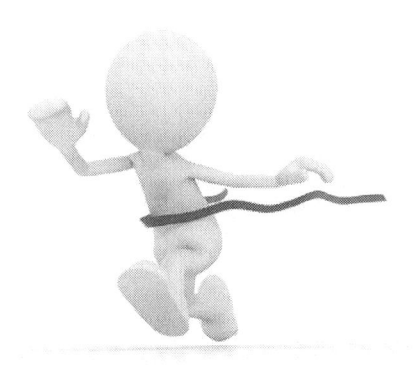

Concussion Recovery

Weekly planner:

Schedule your time for what your brain needs now.

Allow yourself time to recover with naps if and when necessary.

	Mon	Tues	Wed	Thu	Fri	Sat	Sun
6:00 am							
7:00							
8:00							
9:00							
10:00							
11:00							
noon							
1:00 pm							
2:00							
3:00							
4:00							
5:00							
6:00							
7:00							
8:00							
9:00							
10:00							
11:00							
12:00am							

Concussion Recovery

When we start with the final stages of the recovery, it is difficult to know when you are pushing beyond your comfort zone and when you are honoring yourself. Be gentle and kind. Once the mind chatter is gone, listen to your body. It does not lie.

Setting new goals and establishing a new routine takes at least 6 weeks. If you fall off the wagon, dust yourself off and start again. Remember the 10,000 hour rule: it takes 10,000 hours to become an expert. Be gentle and kind on yourself.

Goal setting:
This week I want to accomplish:
1. Walking Normal
2. Talking Normal
3. Migrainy go away — fuck off!

If I am kind to myself and live up to my schedule, I will reward myself with:
1. Sleep
2. Being under foot-talk
3. Work on Nova

Concussion Recovery

This month I am choosing to do:

1. No more of this
2. F-in shit in the beuk
3. _____

This is how I am going to achieve this goal:

1. _____
2. _____
3. _____

I choose to reward myself with:

1. _____
2. _____
3. _____

In 3 months, I choose to accomplish:

1. _____
2. _____
3. _____

Concussion Recovery

This is how I am going to achieve this goal:

1. _____
2. _____
3. _____

I choose to reward myself with:

1. _____
2. _____
3. _____

In the next 6 months, I choose to accomplish:

1. _____
2. _____
3. _____

This is how I am going to achieve this goal:

1. _____
2. _____
3. _____

Concussion Recovery

I choose to reward myself with:

1. _____

2. _____

3. _____

In one year, I choose to:

1. _____

2. _____

3. _____

This is how I am going to achieve this goal:

1. _____

2. _____

3. _____

I choose to reward myself with:

1. _____

2. _____

3. _____

Concussion Recovery

Now, create your dream! Go wild! In 5 years, I am going to have accomplished:

1. _____
2. _____
3. _____

I choose to reward myself with:

1. _____
2. _____
3. _____

What are the gifts and opportunities that you have learned through your ordeal?

1. _____
2. _____
3. _____

Draw a picture of the road you have traveled and where you are now. Congratulations!

Concussion Recovery

Too much fluff - happy, joy
Fa-la-la-

If ones mind is always busy
with clutter - stress - etc
where is the capacity to say
and think - I choose
      I feel
      I am
      Joy Joy
      Happy.
... and lie to yourself ???!

Some of this book is ~~so~~ useful.
From the point of an analytical,
logical, problem solving perspective.
Much is too fluffy, much of
it is common sense. Or
a collection of yoga - mindfulness
self help material readily available
in great abundance, if not too
much.

Concussion Recovery

To try:
    Brain Builders pg 84
    Cross touch
    Crossword
    Word Search

Concussion Recovery

Your brain can be taken from you.

It is yours to reclaim and rebuild.

Appendix B: Bibliography

Balch, Phyllis. Prescription for Nutritional Healing 5th Edition. New York: Penguin Group, c2010

Brennan, Barbara Ann. Hands of Light. New York: Bantam Books, c1987

Bolte Taylor, Jill. My Stroke of Insight. New York: Penguin Books, c2009

Buzan, Tony. Brain Boot Camp. London, England: HarperCollins, c2007

Buzan, Tony. Memory Boot Camp. London, England: HarperCollins, c2010

Caulfield, Timothy. The Cure For Everything! Ontario: Penguin Publishing, c2012

Cloud, Henry, John Townsend. Boundaries. Michigan: Zondervan, c1992

Dennison, Paul and Gail. Brain Gym Teacher's Edition. California: Hearts at Play, c2010

Dennison, Paul and Gail. Brain Gym. California: Edukinesthetics Inc., c2010

Detzler, Robert. Soul Re-Creation: Developing Your Cosmic Potential. Washington: Snohomish, c1999

Doidge, Norman. The Brain that Changes Itself. New York: Penguin Books, c2007

Espiau Wood, Dorothy. The Gems of Excellence. Arizona: Espiau's Circles of Life. c1987

Glenville, Marilyn. Natural Alternatives to Dieting. British Columbia: Whitecap Books, c1999

Hay, Louise. Heal Your Body. California: Hay House, c1988

Concussion Recovery

Hicks, Jerry and Esther. <u>Ask and It is Given</u>. California: Hay House, c2004

Katz, Leonard. <u>Keeping your Brain Alive</u>. New York: Workman, c1999

Murphy, Joseph. <u>The Power of Your Subconscious Mind</u>. New York: Prentice Hall Press, c2008

Norden, Jeanette. <u>Understanding the Brain</u>. Virginia: The Teaching Company, c2007

Pollard, Jimmy. <u>Hurry up and Wait: A Cognitive Care Companion</u>. Pennsylvania: self published, c2008

Silver, Jonathan et all. <u>Textbook of Traumatic Brain Injury</u>. Washington, DC: American Psychiatric Publishing, c2011

Truman, Karol. <u>Feelings Buried Alive Never Die</u>. Utah: Olympus Distributing, c2003

I have been uplifted, informed and inspired by the vast amount of knowledge that I have found on the internet. (Be careful! Do not believe everything that you read!)

My top 5 sites (although I had to leave out many more good ones.):

The Canadian Institute of Health Research: http://www.cihr.ca
Canadian Centre for Disease Control And Prevention: http://www.cdc.gov/TraumaticBrainInjury/
Touted as 'your gateway to information about the brain and brain research', Dana often offers some incredible insights: www.Dana.org

Concussion Recovery

Neurological health charities of Canada:
www.mybrainmatters.ca

Your Canadian online source of the most current and reliable information about spinal cord injury and disease: http://www.spinalcordconnections.ca/

Toronto Rehab researches to maximize life for people living with the effects of disability, illness and aging: www.torontorehab.on.ca /research

Appendix C: Endnotes

[i] Disabled World - Disability News for all the Family: *http://www.disabled-world.com/artman/publish/brain-facts.shtml#ixzz1odkBtNA7*

[ii] *This great blog entry explains how we must continually build our brains.*
http://colinblundell.wordpress.com/2012/01/07/the-brain-begins-to-decline-at-40/

[iii] *www.dana.org*

[iv] *http://www.psychologydegree.net/2009/06/14/25-scientifically-proven-ways-to-make-yourself-smarter/*

[v] *http://www.pickthebrain.com/blog/overcoming-the-loss-of-motivation-that-follows-a-surge-of-productivity/*

[vi] Exercise makes you smarter.
http://blogs.scientificamerican.com/guest-blog/2011/03/07/you-can-increase-your-intelligence-5-ways-to-maximize-your-cognitive-potential/

[vii] Exercise builds new neuron connections.
http://www.dana.org/news/brainwork/detail.aspx?id=7374

[viii] *Strength training helps everyone!*
http://www.nj.gov/health/senior/documents/healthease_directory

[ix] Dr. Doepp is a holistic practitioner who has developed brain mapping and different techniques.
http://www.youtube.com/watch?v=n0Sg6BZAUU8&feature=related

Concussion Recovery

[x] Music grows brains.
http://www.sciencedaily.com/releases/2001/05/010510072912.htm

Made in the USA
Lexington, KY
26 July 2012